GENETICS OF MENTAL DISORDERS

GENETICS OF MENTAL DISORDERS

What Practitioners and Students Need to Know

STEPHEN V. FARAONE
MING T. TSUANG
DEBBY W. TSUANG

THE GUILFORD PRESS
New York   London

© 1999 The Guilford Press
A Division of Guilford Publications, Inc.
72 Spring Street, New York, NY 10012
www.guilford.com

Printed in the United States of America

This book is printed on acid-free paper.

Last digit is print number: 9 8 7 6 5 4 3 2

Library of Congress Cataloging-in-Publication Data
for the hardcover edition:

Faraone, Stephen V.
    Genetics of mental disorders: a guide for students, clinicians,
and researchers / Stephen V. Faraone, Ming T. Tsuang, Debby
W. Tsuang.
        p.   cm.
    Includes bibliographical references and index.
    ISBN 1-57230-479-0 (hard)
    1. Mental illness—Genetic aspects. 2. Medical genetics—
Psychological aspects. I. Tsuang, Ming T. 1931–. II. Tsuang,
Debby W. III. Title.
    [DNLM: 1. Genetic Predisposition to Disease—genetics.
2. Hereditary Diseases—genetics. 3. Mental Disorders—genetics.
4. Psychiatry—methods.   WM 140 F219g 1999]
RC455.4.G4F37 1999
616.89′042—dc21
DNLM/DLC
for Library of Congress   99-13077
                                                                    CIP

ISBN 1-57230-739-0 (paperback)

Acknowledgments

*M*any colleagues have influenced the ideas expressed in this book. Although these are too many to mention, we thank them for their collaborative work on research projects, their free exchange of scientific ideas, and their friendship. We also thank Karen Irwin, Lisa Gabel, BA, and Molly Wamble, BFA, for assistance in manuscript preparation.

About the Authors

Stephen V. Faraone, a clinical psychologist, is Associate Professor in the Department of Psychiatry at Harvard Medical School at the Massachusetts Mental Health Center. He is also Director of Pediatric Psychopharmacology Research at Massachusetts General Hospital. Dr. Faraone is Co-Editor of the journal *Neuropsychiatric Genetics* and Statistical Section Editor of the *Journal of Child and Adolescent Psychopharmacology*. He also serves as a member of the Panel of Biostatistical and Methodology Consultants for the *Journal of the American Academy of Child and Adolescent Psychiatry*. At Harvard Medical School Dr. Faraone is principal investigator on several National Institutes of Health grants designed to clarify the nature and causes of attention-deficit hyperactivity disorder and is coinvestigator on several studies aimed at clarifying the genetics of schizophrenia and of substance abuse. The author of over 300 journal articles, editorials, chapters, and books, he was the eighth highest producer of high-impact papers in psychiatry from 1990 to 1999, as determined by the Institute for Scientific Information (*Science,* 2000, Vol. 288, p. 959).

Ming T. Tsuang is internationally known for his studies of the psychiatric epidemiology, nosology, and genetics of schizophrenia and mood disorders. Subsequent to the award of his MD degree from National Taiwan University, he earned his PhD in psychiatry at the Institute of Psychiatry, University of London, and his DSc in psychiatric genetics and epidemiology from the Faculty of Science, University of London. Currently, Dr. Tsuang is Stanley Cobb Professor of Psychiatry at Harvard Medical School; Superintendent and Head, Harvard Department of Psychiatry at the Massachusetts Mental Health Center; and Director of the Harvard Institute of Psychiatric Epidemiology and Genetics jointly sponsored by the Harvard Schools of Medicine and Public Health. He is also Chairman of the Veterans Affairs Cooperative Linkage Study of Schizophrenia at the Brockton/West Roxbury VA Medical Center. In addition to being Editor of the journal *Neuropsychiatric Genetics* and a member of numerous editorial boards, he continues to pursue epidemiological and genetic studies of schizophrenia, mood disorders, and substance use disorders. He is also a member of the National Advisory Mental Health Council of the U.S. Department of Health and Human Services. In recognition of his distinguished clinical and research career, Dr. Tsuang was elected Member, Institute of Medicine, National Academy of Sciences, and is a member of the Academia Sinica of Taiwan. He was also elected Fellow in the American College of Psychiatrists and the Royal College of Psychiatrists of the United Kingdom. For his contributions to psychiatric research, Dr. Tsuang was awarded the Rema Lapouse Award for Mental Health Epidemiology, presented by the Mental Health, Epidemiology, and Statistics Sections of the American Public Health Association; the Stanley Dean Award for Basic Research in Schizophrenia, American College of Psychiatrists; the Lifetime Achievement Award, International Society of Psychiatric Genetics; and the Gold Medal Award, Society of Biological Psychiatry.

Debby W. Tsuang received her MD and Master's of Science (Psychiatric Epidemiology) from the University of Iowa. She completed her geriatric psychiatry fellowship at the University of Washington, with an emphasis on genetics of dementia. She is currently Assistant Professor in the Departments of Psychiatry and Behavioral Sciences and Epidemiology at the University of Washington. She is also a research investigator in the Veterans Affairs Mental Illness Research, Clinical and Education Center (MIRECC), based at the VA Puget Sound Health Care System. Dr. Tsuang serves as an ad hoc reviewer for several journals in geriatric and general psychiatry and medical genetics. Her research focuses on the genetics of Alzheimer disease, Huntington disease and schizophrenia.

Contents

FIGURES AND TABLES   xiii

CHAPTER 1   INTRODUCTION   1

What Is Psychiatric Genetics   2
Clinical Uses of Psychiatric Genetics   4
Genes, Environment, and the Genesis of Psychopathology   7
The Chain of Psychiatric Genetic Research   11

CHAPTER 2   THE BASICS: EPIDEMIOLOGIC FOUNDATIONS   15
             OF PSYCHIATRIC GENETICS

Is a Disorder Familial?: The Case–Control Family Study   16
   Evaluating Family Studies 21
Is the Disorder Genetic?: Twin Studies   29
   Partitioning Genetic and Environmental Sources of Illness 32
   Evaluating Twin Studies 37
Is the Disorder Genetic?: Adoption Studies   39
   Evaluating Adoption Studies 42
Summary: Epidemiologic Foundations of Psychiatric Genetics   43

CHAPTER 3   VARIATIONS ON A THEME: CAUSAL   46
             AND CLINICAL HETEROGENEITY

Can We Define Genetic and Nongenetic Subtypes?   50
Are There Genetic Variants of the Disorder?   55

How Do We Identify Genetic Spectrum Disorders? 58
Spectrum Conditions for Other Disorders 61

What Are the Neurobiologic Correlates of Genetic Predisposition?   63

Do Two or More Disorders Share Familial Causal Factors?   70

Why Do Two Disorder Co-Occur   74

How Do We Show Developmental Continuity Between Disorders   89
of Children and Adults?

CHAPTER 4   MATHEMATICAL MODELS OF INHERITANCE   93

Modes of Genetic Transmission   94
Single-Gene Inheritance 94
Oligogenic Inheritance 100
Multifactoral Polygenic Inheritance 101

Segregation Analysis: Determining the Mode of Transmission   106
Overview of Mathematical Modeling 107
Path Analysis 109

Obstacles to Establishing the Mode of Inheritance   112

CHAPTER 5   MOLECULAR GENETICS AND MENTAL ILLNESS   115

Biologic Background   117

DNA Markers for Linkage Analysis   124

Statistical Methods for Linkage Analysis   126
The Affected Pedigree Member Method of Linkage Analysis 129
The Lod Score Method of Linkage Analysis 131
Guidelines for Interpreting Linkage Results 133
Examples of Linkage Analysis 134

Association Studies   136
Population-Based Association Studies 136
Family-Based Association Studies 140

The Search for Disease Mechanisms   143
Finding Mutations That Cause Disease 143
Types of Mutations 144
Cytogenetic Abnormalities and Psychiatric Disorders 146
Animal Models of Human Disorders 152
Disease Genes and Environmental Mechanisms 155

CHAPTER 6   CLINICAL APPLICATIONS OF PSYCHIATRIC GENETICS   159

Genetic Counselling for Psychiatric Disorders   160
Stages of Genetic Counseling 160
A Case Study 183

Implications for Diagnosis and Treatment　　　　　　188
　　Family-Based Diagnosis 188
　　Fighting Therapeutic Nihilism 191
　　Facilitating Treatment 193

CHAPTER 7　　THE FUTURE OF PSYCHIATRIC GENETICS　　196

The Promise of New Technologies　　　　　　　　197
　　Molecular Genetics: The Human Genome Project 197
　　A Clinical Nosology for Psychiatric Genetics 199
The Future of Predictive Genetic Testing　　　　　206
　　Presymptomatic Genetic Testing 206
　　Lessons from Predictive Testing in Huntington Disease 209
The Future of Mental Health Treatment　　　　　213
　　Early Identification and Prevention of Disorders 213
　　Medical Interventions for Genetic Defects 219
Ethical Issues for the Science and Practice of Psychiatric Genetics　222
　　The Shadow of Eugenics 222
　　Ethical Issues for Genetic Testing 225
　　Informed Consent: The Cornerstone of Ethical Research and Practice
　　　231
　　Ethical Issues for Gene Therapy 231

GLOSSARY　　　　　　　　　　　　　　　　235

READINGS IN PSYCHIATRIC GENETICS　　　　　　247

INTERNET RESOURCES FOR PSYCIATRIC GENETICS　　257

INDEX　　　　　　　　　　　　　　　　　　260

Figures and Tables

FIGURES

FIGURE 1.1	How genes and environment lead to illness and spectrum conditions	8
FIGURE 1.2	Developmental sequence of pathophysiology	9
FIGURE 2.1	Family study of attention-deficit/hyperactivity disorder	18
FIGURE 2.2	Lifetime prevalence of schizophrenia by degree of genetic relationship to a schizophrenic patient	20
FIGURE 2.3	Multifactorial model of vulnerability	31
FIGURE 2.4	Sources of variance from twin studies of mood disorders	33
FIGURE 2.5	Effects of genes and environment on antisocial traits	34
FIGURE 2.6	Bipolar disorder and depression among the adoptive and biologic parents and bipolar and normal adoptees	41
FIGURE 3.1	Causal and clinical heterogeneity	47
FIGURE 3.2	Genetic subtypes of schizophrenia	54
FIGURE 3.3	Multifactorial model of vulnerability	56
FIGURE 3.4	Mixed multifactorial model of vulnerability	57
FIGURE 3.5	Neuropsychologic functioning among the nonpsychotic relatives of schizophrenic patients	65
FIGURE 3.6	Summary test scores for relatives of schizophrenic patients and controls	66

FIGURE 3.7   Structural brain abnormalities in a relative of a   67
               schizophrenic patient as illustrated by brain slices
               imaged by MRI

FIGURE 3.8   Adjusted volumes in selected brain regions   68

FIGURE 3.9   Studies examining the familial link between bipolar   71
               disorder and major depression

FIGURE 3.10   Prevalence of schizophrenia and mood disorders in   73
               relatives of schizophrenic and mood-disordered
               patients

FIGURE 3.11   Increased odds of having other disorders for   76
               subjects with major depressive disorder

FIGURE 3.12   Schematic pedigree of comorbid disorders   79

FIGURE 3.13   Prevalence of ADHD and LD among relatives of   81
               ADHD, ADHD + LD, and control probands

FIGURE 3.14   Independent transmission of ADHD and LD   81

FIGURE 3.15   Nonrandom mating between ADHD and LD   82
               parents

FIGURE 3.16   ADHD among children of depressed and control   84
               parents

FIGURE 3.17   Depression among relatives of ADHD and control   84
               children

FIGURE 3.18   Depression among relatives of ADHD probands   85
               with and without major depressive disorder (MDD)

FIGURE 3.19   CD among relatives of ADHD and control children   86

FIGURE 3.20   Patterns of familial transmission predicted by   88
               models of psychiatric comorbidity

FIGURE 3.21   Anxiety disorders among children of panic   92
               disorder and control patients

FIGURE 4.1A   A pedigree of a family with autosomal dominant   96
               disease

FIGURE 4.1B   Transmission of an autosomal dominant trait   96

FIGURE 4.2A   A pedigree of a family with an autosomal recessive   98
               trait

FIGURE 4.2B   Transmission of an autosomal recessive trait   98

FIGURE 4.3A   A pedigree of a family with an X-linked recessive   99
               trait

FIGURE 4.3B   Transmission of an X-linked recessive trait   99

FIGURE 4.4   Hypothetical frequency distribution of a   102
              continuous variable (height): one genetic locus

FIGURE 4.5   Frequency distribution of a continuous variable: 103
              two genetic loci

FIGURE 4.6   Genetic liability among first-, second-, and third- 105
              degree relatives, illustrating differences in genetic
              liability between affected individuals and
              individuals in the general population

FIGURE 4.7   Two-threshold model for major depressive disorder 106
              and bipolar mood disorder

FIGURE 4.8   A path diagram demonstrating contributions of   110
              various genetic and environmental effects to a
              phenotype

FIGURE 4.9   A twin-family model for twins and their parents   111
              applied to alcoholism

FIGURE 4.10   A pedigree of a family with mitochondrial   114
              inheritance

FIGURE 5.1   Schematic representation of a chromosome   118

FIGURE 5.2   Schematic representation of a gene and its protein 119
              product

FIGURE 5.3   A schematic representation of a single crossover in 121
              a chromosome pair

FIGURE 5.4   Genetic marker status from linkage analysis of an 127
              autosomal dominant condition

FIGURE 5.5   A normal female karyotype   147

FIGURE 5.6   Representation of the human genome, consisting   148
              of 22 pairs of autosomes and 1 pair of sex
              chromosomes

FIGURE 5.7   Schematic representation of chromosome 6, with   149
              delineation of specific arm, region, sample bands,
              genetic markers, and genes

FIGURE 6.1   Common pedigree symbols, definitions, and   168
              abbreviations

FIGURE 6.2   Pedigree line definitions   169

FIGURE 6.3   Weighing risks and benefits in genetic counseling 180

FIGURE 6.4   Hypothetical pedigree   184

TABLES

TABLE 1.1   Chain of Psychiatric Genetic Research   11

TABLE 1.2   Examples of Diseases with Known Genetic Loci   13

TABLE 2.1   Three Basic Genetic Epidemiologic Designs   16

TABLE 2.2   Procedures to Improve the Family History Method   27

TABLE 2.3   Examples of Less Stringent Diagnostic Criteria   28

TABLE 2.4   Family Study vs. Family History Method   29

TABLE 2.5   Disentangling Genes from Environment in Twin   32
             Studies

TABLE 2.6   Types of Adoption Studies   39

TABLE 3.1   Questions and Answers for Family, Twin, and   49
             Adoption Studies

TABLE 3.2   Criteria for Classifying a Trait as a Spectrum   59
             Condition of a Disorder

TABLE 3.3   Examples of Spectrum Conditions   62

TABLE 3.4   Possible Causes of Psychiatric Comorbidity   77

TABLE 5.1   Lod Scores for Linkage of Alzheimer Disease to   135
             DNA Markers on Chromosome 14

TABLE 5.2   APOE Genotypes and Allele Frequencies in the   139
             Community Sample Cases and Controls

TABLE 5.3   Ecogenetic Patterns of Gene–Environment   156
             Interaction

TABLE 6.1   Stages of Genetic Counseling   162

TABLE 6.2   Theoretical Recurrence Risks for Multifactorial   172
             Polygenic Mental Disorders

TABLE 7.1   Measurement/Genetic Level Classification   201
             Outcomes

TABLE 7.2   Examples of Diseases Having Commercially   206
             Available Genetic Tests for Presymptomatic or
             Prenatal Testing

1

Introduction

For every complex problem there is a simple solution which is wrong.

—GEORGE BERNARD SHAW

*I*f you are neither schooled in genetics nor familiar with the arcane language of biologic psychiatry, the phrase "psychiatric genetics" conjures up intimidating images. To some, psychiatric genetics threatens us with a mindless biologic determinism that views personalities, cognitive structures, and psychopathology as the predestined products of the genetic factories in our cells. In this view, psychiatric genetics is a handmaiden to psychopharmacology; together, the two perpetuate a simplistic biological paradigm that would explain mental illness without referring to learning, family interaction, psychologic processes, or other nonbiologic phenomena that may detour human development from its ideal path.

To others, psychiatric genetics casts the dark shadow of eugenics, a political view that uses genetic knowledge to dictate health care options, reproductive rights, or even the right to life itself. Should eugenics become popular with politicians—as it had been in Nazi Germany—it could reduce individuals to genetic types. These types could be used by health and life insurance companies to discriminate against people who carry disease-predisposing genes. Worse, the discovery of genetic types could be used as a political tool by a genetic elite who would justify discrimination, sterilization, or euthanasia against people whose genes forebode a life of mental illness.

1

To us, psychiatric genetics provides a source of hope for us and our patients. It promises that the causes of mental illness will be discovered, that more efficacious treatments can be developed, and that—someday—the tragedy of mental illness can be prevented by intervening prior to its onset. To be sure, psychiatric genetics poses clinical, moral, and political dilemmas, all of which need to be explored and considered by scientists, clinicians, legislators, and patients.

In this book, we will provide you with the facts you will need to make informed clinical and ethical decisions in the not-too-distant future when information about genetic risk will be available to you and your patients. We will show you the tools of psychiatric genetics, explain how they work, and discuss what research has found. But before diving into these details we will offer a broad overview of our science and employ it to address some misconceptions about the profession. After reading this chapter you should have a general idea of what psychiatric genetics is, what it is not, and how it might prove useful to you in clinical practice. You will see that the inheritance of mental illness poses complex problems and that scientists are uncovering the complex solutions you will need to make informed clinical decisions.

WHAT IS PSYCHIATRIC GENETICS?

We mental health practitioners form a diverse group, having many theoretical orientations and therapeutic approaches to the mentally ill. Yet as a group, we all agree on several key principles. Among these is the idea that families play a leading role in the genesis and expression of psychopathology—the signs and symptoms of mental illness. Whether you read the psychoanalytic papers of Sigmund Freud, the research papers of contemporary learning theorists, or the manuals of family therapists, the family emerges as a focal point for understanding the causes, diagnosis, and treatment of mental disorders.

The nearly universal belief that families influence the mental health of their members is an axiom of psychiatric genetics. Indeed, the family is its basic unit of analysis. Actually, the name "psychiatric genetics" is shorthand for "psychiatric genetic epidemiology," a fact that will be useful in explaining the multidisciplinary origin of our science. Some readers may be surprised to find the word "epidemiology" in this book. After all, epidemiologists usually concern themselves with explaining the distribution and determinants of disease by exposures to environmental factors. This leads naturally to the goal of finding environmental risk factors that cause disease. Geneticists, in contrast, are often thought to conduct experimental studies that strictly control the environment in order to eliminate its effects on the genetic pathway to the expression of traits. Put simply, the genetic experiment views the environment as mere "noise" that makes it difficult to observe the effects of genes; classic epidemiology reverses the roles of genes and environment.

In contrast to these extremes, genetic epidemiology, as defined by Newton Morton, is "a science that deals with causes, distribution, and control of disease in groups of relatives and with inherited causes of disease in populations." Genetic epidemiologists examine the pattern of illness within families with the goal of finding genetic *and* environmental causes of illness. Thus, psychiatric genetics considers both genetic and environmental risk factors—and their interaction—to be on an equal footing.

This definition of psychiatric genetics is at odds with simplistic notions about genetic determinism. In fact, as we shall describe in more detail later, psychiatric genetics has provided some of the strongest evidence that the environment plays a causal role in the expression of psychiatric illness. Most notable in this regard are studies of identical twins. These show that, for most psychiatric disorders, a person can be free of illness *even if his or her genetically identical twin is ill*. For example, in the case of schizophrenia, the identical twin of a schizophrenic patient has only a 50 percent chance of ever developing schizophrenia. Why is one twin ill with a devastating disease while the other lives a normal life? We do not know for sure, but a good guess is that, although both twins harbor the genes for schizophrenia, one was exposed to an environmental trigger, the other was not. Such differences between identical twins point to the influence of environmental factors in the causation of psychiatric disorders.

> **Key Point:** Psychiatric geneticists do not pit nature against nurture. Instead, they seek to learn how both work together to cause mental illness.

So, it is best to view psychiatric genetics as a methodology—as a scientific toolbox that we and our colleagues use to understand why disorders occur in some family members but not in others. Most assuredly, this discipline rests on a biological foundation: deoxyribonucleic acid (DNA). As the building block of genes, DNA is the source of genetic transmission; within the cells of the developing fetus it contains instructions for the development of the body, including the central nervous system, which plays a certain role in the causation and expression of mental illness.

But genes do not act in isolation from other genes or from a person's psychologic or physical environment. Think of genes as actors and the environment as their stage. Together they tell the story of human development. As psychiatric geneticists watch the play of psychopathology, they seek to identify the actors and learn how their behavior changes with the surrounding scene.

CLINICAL USES OF PSYCHIATRIC GENETICS

As Chapter 6 discusses in detail, psychiatric genetics has several uses for the mental health practitioner. Paramount among these is family-based diagnosis. In standard practice, we diagnose patients by asking them and their significant others about the signs and symptoms of psychopathology. By noting how these signs correspond to the categories provided by the diagnostic manual, we formulate a diagnosis. With the advent of structured diagnostic criteria (such as those in the fourth edition of the *Diagnostic and Statistical Manual of Mental Disorders* [DSM-IV] of the American Psychiatric Association) this standard diagnostic procedure has become sufficiently reliable and valid to be of use in formulating treatment plans.

Yet any working clinician knows that diagnoses are not always clear: patients may be poor reporters, records from prior mental health contacts may not be available, the patient may be in the early phases of a disorder that cannot be identified. In such cases, family-based diagnosis can be useful. The method is straightforward. We simply ask the patient, and other family members, about the family's psychiatric history.

As a hypothetical example, imagine a young adult patient who, after a year of gradual decline in her ability to socialize and to perform competently at work, arrives in your office with symptoms of mania, but also shows psychotic signs that raise the suspicion of a schizophrenic disorder. In isolation, this patient's diagnosis may not be clear until the passage of time clarifies its course. In making a provisional diagnosis, you might resolve this ambiguity by learning more about the psychiatric history of the family. For example, if you learn that the patient's sister has been diagnosed with bipolar disorder, your confidence in a diagnosis of bipolar disorder for the patient would increase. If the sister had been diagnosed as paranoid schizophrenic, that disorder would certainly deserve serious consideration.

> **Clinical Tip:** We can learn much about the psychiatric condition of our patients by knowing which disorders affect their family members.

Of course, family-based diagnosis cannot replace the careful documentation of psychopathology that will eventually clarify ambiguous diagnoses. But when diagnostic data are lean and clinical decisions must be made, knowledge of psychiatric genetics can lead to more accurate diagnoses. In some cases, the benefit to the patient could be substantial. The differential diagnosis of schizophrenia and bipolar disorder is paradigmatic. For both disorders, research suggests that early pharmacologic treatment can mitigate the course of illness. The basic idea is that untreated episodes of illness harm the brain in a manner that makes it more susceptible to subsequent episodes, and thus to a chronic course of illness and disability. Consequently, the correct treatment at the first onset of symptoms may reduce the patient's degree of lifelong suffering. Because family-based diagnosis can clarify ambiguous diagnoses, it can help patients by improving the accuracy of early treatment decisions.

In addition to facilitating accurate diagnoses, knowledge of psychiatric genetics will help clinicians incorporate genetic counseling into their therapeutic practice. A depressed patient, concerned about his children, may ask about their chance of becoming depressed. The patient's younger sister, having seen her brother suffer the harrowing consequences of severe depression, may wonder if she too will fall prey to the disorder. Such concerns may lead to direct questions about the risk of illness for which direct answers are usually possible and frequently reassuring.

For some family members, concerns about risk may lurk as latent anxieties, leading to maladaptive behavior and psychological distress. From reports in the popular press, family members may form misconceptions about risk which, if not corrected, may worsen family functioning. Notably, the last decade has seen news reports about genes for schizophrenia, bipolar disorder, and attention-deficit/hyperactivity disorder, along with media discussions of breakthroughs in genetics (indeed, as we write this chapter, the media has reported on successful attempts to clone sheep and monkeys).

As molecular genetic technology accelerates, our patients and their families will be increasingly exposed to genetic information. We can help them process this information—and use it for effective therapeutic change—but only if we understand what has been discovered, how it was discovered, and how certain we can be of the results. Providing a framework for such knowledge is a goal of this book.

> **Key Point:** Molecular genetic studies will lead to breakthroughs in diagnosis, treatment, and primary preven-

> tion. You can expect many questions from patients and their families.

Paradoxically, psychiatric genetics can also help therapists defeat what Paul Meehl called "therapeutic nihilism," the belief that only biologic treatments can help persons afflicted with "genetic" disorders. Consider an anxiety-ridden patient who reads in the morning paper that her fear and angst are distal messages from neurons foiled by faulty genetic instructions. She may well wonder whether talking through her problems, or contemplating her past, or doing her behavior therapy assignments can have any effect on such a deeply rooted problem. In fact, they can, but it would take an empathic therapist who understands psychiatric genetic data to show that this is so. Understanding psychiatric genetics will help therapists transform the turmoil induced by the latest genetic news into productive energy that can be harnessed for therapeutic change.

The most powerful clinical use of psychiatric genetics is still a possibility: the primary prevention of mental illness. In the coming decades—as disease genes are discovered, their mutations catalogued, and their aberrant products described—the genetic architecture of mental illness will emerge as the intricate edifice that it must be. This knowledge may someday make the impossible routine: we will have the ability to identify which children are and are not at very high genetic risk for mental illness.

This ability to predict will set the stage for powerful psychiatric genetic studies of environmental causes of illness. Currently, studies of environmental causes must examine heterogeneous samples of people at high, medium, and low risk for illness, without knowing who fits into which category. This would be expected to produce ambiguous results. For example, if we were to study the effects of family conflict on depression among a random sample of adolescents, we might find no effect. If we focused our study on children of depressed mothers, that effect might increase, but would still be ambiguous because only a fraction of these children will carry the genetic predisposition for depression. But when future discoveries make it possible to study children who all have the genetic predisposition for depression (as determined by assays of their DNA), we may be able to discover those features of the environment that trigger genes for depression or prevent their expression.

A comprehensive understanding of how environmental triggers lead to mental illness should set the stage for preventive trials aimed at mitigating their effects on genetically susceptible children. Such trials could use psychologic therapies to reduce adverse family interactions or teach children coping skills. They might also use psychopharmacologic agents that ameliorate the biological weaknesses that genes have wrought in the brain. Moreover, although the idea of "gene therapy" sounds like science fiction, the direct modification of genes may someday correct mutations before they have a chance to detour the normal path of brain development.

GENES, ENVIRONMENT, AND THE GENESIS OF PSYCHOPATHOLOGY

To help you understand what will follow, this section provides a theoretical framework that describes—in broad strokes—how we view the causes of psychopathology. This framework is offered as a set of organizing principles, not as a definitive guide. Nevertheless, with some exceptions, it should be applicable to most mental disorders.

We will begin our foray into etiologic theory with a conclusion: *most mental disorders exhibit complex inheritance.* If you could retain only a single lesson from this book, the concept of complex inheritance would serve you well. This principle posits that, unlike Huntington disease, which follows a simple and inexorable genetic rule (inheriting one copy of the mutant gene leads to certain illness, disability, and death), the transmission of psychiatric disorders most likely requires the interaction of several genes and environmental factors that transmit a predisposition to illness but do not always lead to disease. Thus, some genetically vulnerable people will be normal, others will have mild psychopathology, and still others will have neurobiologic abnormalities of unknown clinical significance.

> **Key Point:** There is no single genetic switch that when flipped causes some psychiatric disorder. The causes of mental illnesses are complex, requiring many interacting genes and environmental factors.

We use the term "spectrum conditions" to indicate the full range of effects that can be caused by a set of disease genes. A well-studied example is schizotypal personality, a spectrum condition for schizophrenia. A person with schizotypal personality has a relatively mild condition that includes features such as magical ideation, odd speech, and social withdrawal that are similar to but less serious than the signs and symptoms of schizophrenia. In Chapter 3 we will provide more examples of spectrum conditions and show how psychiatric genetic research designs clarify their clinical implications.

Figure 1.1 provides a graphic view of how genes combine with the environment to cause disease and spectrum conditions. The horizontal axis of Figure 1.1 corresponds to the level of genetic predisposition that is caused by a set of genes. The vertical axis indexes the level of environmental risk factors to which a person is exposed. The solid line demarcates the threshold of combined genetic and environmental risk required for a person to become ill.

Persons who have high levels of genetic and environmental risk (such as Person A in the figure) will fall in the region labeled "Full Disorder." Those with moderately high levels (e.g., Person B) will fall in the region bounded by the broken and solid lines; they will have spectrum conditions. Person C, and others with low values of genetic and environmental risk, will not be at risk for either the full disorder or its milder spectrum abnormalities. The figure implies that both environmental and genetic risk factors are needed to trigger illness. It is possible, however, that for some disorders a high enough dose either of adverse environmental risk factors or of predisposing genes would be sufficient.

We must also consider the developmental sequence of gene expression from conception through birth and from childhood through adulthood. Figure 1.2 shows a simplified developmental model that will apply (at least in part) to many psychiatric disorders. The top of the Figure defines the starting point of psychopathology: the set of disease-predisposing genes that is determined at conception. The flawed blue-

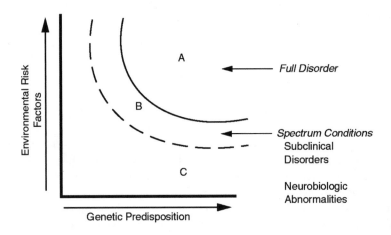

FIGURE 1.1. How genes and environment lead to illness and spectrum conditions.

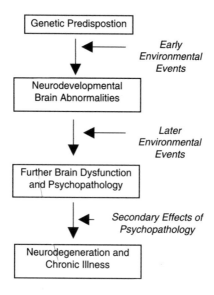

FIGURE 1.2. Developmental sequence of pathophysiology.

print dictated by these genes builds a brain that is susceptible to mental illness.

The exact nature of this brain dysfunction is unknown. Perhaps key connections between brain cells are not made. It is also possible that the chemicals that brain cells use to communicate with one another are not produced in the correct quantities or that the cell structures needed for effective communication are malformed. Whatever the underlying pathophysiology, this aberrant brain circuitry is only a beginning.

The next step in the pathophysiologic chain occurs when the brain is exposed to "early environmental events" as indicated in the top section of the figure. By "early," we mean while the child is still a fetus or at some other time close to birth. Many such events have been implicated in the genesis of psychiatric illness. These include viral infection and complications of either pregnancy or delivery. Thus, the top portion of the figure underscores a key point: *the interplay between genes and environment can occur even before the birth of the child.*

> **Clinical Tip:** Figure 1.2 shows how adverse environmental events cause illness. But it also implies that corrective environmental events (e.g., psychosocial therapies) can intervene

> in the causal pathway. Showing this figure to patients and explaining its meaning can help them understand why psychosocial therapies are helpful for mental illnesses that are described as diseases of the brain.

The next section of the figure indicates that genes and early environmental events create neurodevelopmental brain abnormalities and spectrum conditions. *Neurodevelopmental* means that, because the brain has been affected during its development, it is never completely normal. This contrasts with other conditions such as brain damage caused by head injury, in which a normal brain has been made abnormal by an external event.

Figure 1.2 also shows that our model allows for the possibility that later environmental events combine with neurodevelopmental anomalies to cause illness. This means that when an already compromised CNS is exposed to adverse environments, further brain dysfunction occurs and psychopathology ensues. Examples of adverse events include drug abuse and stressful home environment.

Our developmental model of psychopathology also postulates possible secondary effects of psychopathology, as indicated at the bottom of the figure. This allows for the possibility that, rather than remaining static, the brain impairments underlying psychopathology can worsen over time. We use the term "neurodegeneration" to indicate that the brain (or neural) pathways involved in the disorder degenerate due to secondary effects of psychopathology.

Neurodegeneration may occur through several pathways. For example, psychopathology could lead to disruptions in interpersonal relations, occupational performance, or other areas of functioning. Through the biologic mechanisms controlling social learning, these effects could modify relevant brain systems and create a downward spiral of worsening psychopathology and chronic impairment. A less speculative example relevant to psychotic syndromes such as schizophrenia or bipolar disorder is the idea that psychotic episodes are toxic to the brain. This theory posits that when psychosis occurs, it permanently scars the brain in a manner that increases the probability that the patient will have additional episodes. This phenomenon is sometimes called "kindling," which implies that a small and relatively innocuous psychotic "fire" in the brain now can lead to a larger, disabling psychotic "firestorm" in the future. Evidence for kindling comes from studies of schizophrenic patients showing that longer durations of untreated psychosis lead to poorer outcomes. These studies have led to clinical programs aimed at identifying and treating psychotic episodes as soon as possible.

Figures 1.1 and 1.2 are but brief sketches of the phenomena that psychiatric genetics seeks to explain and control for the benefit of patients. To do so, the profession has developed a systematic approach to the study of mental disorders in families: the chain of psychiatric genetic research.

THE CHAIN OF PSYCHIATRIC GENETIC RESEARCH

Work in psychiatric genetics tends to follow a series of questions in a logical progression. We call this sequence "the chain of psychiatric genetic research." As Table 1.1 shows, we first ask, "Is the disorder familial?", that is, does it run in families? This stage of research often starts with an astute clinician who notices that the relatives of patients with a certain disorder frequently have the disorder as well. Such observations motivate researchers to pursue systematic family studies. As we show in Chapter 2, these provide us with a relatively simple method to determine if a disorder is truly familial.

Of course, "familial" and "genetic" are not synonymous. Disorders can run in families for many reasons: genes, cultural transmission, shared environmental adversity, and so forth. Thus, after establishing that a disorder runs in families, the psychiatric geneticist asks: "What are the relative contributions of genes and environment as causes of mental illness?" To answer this question, we need to study special types of family relationships and use sophisticated mathematical methods. The two most useful types of families for our purposes are those with twins and those with adopted children. In Chapter 2 we show how

TABLE 1.1. Chain of Psychiatric Genetic Research

Questions	Methods
Is the disorder familial?	Family study
What are the relative contributions of genes and environment?	Twin and adoption studies
Are psychiatric disorders genetically heterogeneous?	Family, twin, and adoption studies
What is the mode of transmission?	Segregation analysis
Where is (are) the gene (genes) located?	Linkage and association studies
What are the mechanisms of disease prevention?	Epidemiologic and treatment studies

these methods can parse the etiology of disorders into three components: genes, shared environment (e.g., low social class), and nonshared environment (e.g., a traumatic experience).

In addition to answering these basic questions concerning psychiatric genetics, the triad of family, twin, and adoption studies can answer many questions about the heterogeneity of psychiatric disorders.
These studies can assess two types of nonuniformity in the expression
of mental illness: causal heterogeneity and clinical heterogeneity.
Studies of causal heterogeneity ask if subtypes of a disorder have different genetic or nongenetic causes. They also ask if the causes of one disorder also affect the expression of other disorders. Studies of clinical
heterogeneity ask if the genetic predisposition to a disorder can lead to
other disorders or outcomes besides the disorder of interest. We discuss issues of heterogeneity in Chapter 3.

Having established the relative contributions of these three components, the psychiatric geneticist then asks: "How is the disease transmitted from generation to generation?" Thus, research will attempt to
determine if one gene causes the disorder or if several work in combination to increase the risk for illness. Mathematical methods can also
determine if cultural transmission occurs and if such transmission varies with features of the family such as the sex and age of its members.
The method for examining these issues, segregation analysis, is discussed in Chapter 4.

> **Key Point:** No one study proves or disproves any-
> thing. Scientists require a pattern of converging evi-
> dence from multiple studies before they can
> reasonably conclude that genes play a role in causing
> a disease.

If twin or adoption research has established that genes play a substantial role in causing illness, the psychiatric geneticist will be keen on
locating these genes. By tracking the coinheritance of DNA segments
and disease in families, the psychiatric geneticist uses a combination of
molecular genetic and statistical technologies to localize genes and
identify mutations that predispose to mental illness. Table 1.2 lists examples of diseases for which one or more causative genes have been
found. From this we can infer that the ability of geneticists to find
genes is well established. As we shall see in Chapter 5, molecular genetic methods have already discovered genes for one psychiatric disorder: Alzheimer disease. We will also discuss why progress for other
psychiatric disorders has been slower and why we believe breakthroughs are on the horizon. As you will see, these breakthroughs will

TABLE 1.2. Examples of Diseases with Known Genetic Loci

Aarskog-Scott syndrome	Huntington disease (chorea)
Achondroplasia	Hyperexplexia
Adenomatous polyposis coli	Hypophosphatemic rickets
Adrenoleukodystrophy, X-linked	Kallman syndrome
Agammaglobulinemia, X-linked	Limb-girdle muscular dystrophy
Alzheimer disease	Long QT syndrome
Amyotrophic lateral sclerosis	Lowe oculocerebrorenal syndrome
Anhidrotic ectodermal dysplasia	Machado-Joseph disease
Aniridia	McLeod syndrome
Ataxia telangiectasia	Menkes disease
Barth syndrome	Miller-Dieker lissencephaly
Basal cell nevus syndrome	Multiple endocrine neoplasia, type 2a
Bloom syndrome	Myotonic dystrophy
Breast cancer, type 1	Myotubular myopathy 1, X-linked
Breast cancer, type 2	Neurofibromatosis, type 1
Chedial-Higashi syndrome	Neurofibromatosis, type 2
Chondrodysplasia punctata	Norrie disease
Choroideremia	Obesity
Chronic granulomatous disease	Ocular albinism
Congenital adrenal hyperplasia	Polycystic kidney disease, type 1
Cystic fibrosis	Polycystic kidney disease, type 2
Dementia, hereditary multi-infarct	Progressive myoclonic epilepsy
Denatorubral pallidoluysianatrophy	Retinitis pigmentosa, X-linked
Diabetes of the young, maturity onset	Retinoblastoma
Diastrophic dysplasia	Rieger syndrome, type 1
Duchenne muscular dystrophy	Simpson-Golabi-Behmel syndrome
Emery-Dreifuss muscular dystrophy	Spinal muscular atrophy
Epidermolytic palmoplantarkeratoderma	Spinocerebe llar ataxia 2
Fanconi anemia A	Spinocerebellar ataxia 1
Fragile-X syndrome	Thomsen disease
Friedreich ataxia	Treacher Collins syndrome
Glycerol kinase deficiency	Tuberous sclerosis
Gonadal dysgenesis	von Hippel-Lindau syndrome
Hemochromatosis	Waardenburg syndrome
Hereditary multiple exostoses, type 1	Werner syndrome
Hereditary multiple exostoses, type 2	Wilms tumor
Hereditary nonpolyposis colon cancer	Wilson disease
Hermansky-Pudlak syndrome	Wiskott-Aldrich syndrome

Note. Adapted from National Human Genome Research Institute web site http:/genome.nhgri.gov/clone/

shed much light on both the genetic and the environmental mechanisms that cause mental illness.

In Chapter 6, we will show how your growing knowledge of psychiatric genetics can be used in clinical settings. We first discuss genetic counseling, which provides principles to help clinicians communicate genetic risks to patients and their families. Then we will show how psychiatric genetics can improve diagnosis and treatment.

We end this book by speculating about the future of psychiatric genetics. Chapter 7 will discuss possible answers to many questions: What is the Human Genome Project and how will it stimulate new molecular genetic technologies? How can improvements in psychologic and psychiatric measurements speed gene discovery? Will the discovery of mental illness genes lead to genetic tests and new treatments for mental disorders? What are the ethical challenges that clinicians, patients, families, and society will face after mental illness genes have been discovered?

2

The Basics:
Epidemiologic Foundations
of Psychiatric Genetics

*If you have built castles in the air, your work need not be lost;
that is where they should be. Now put the foundations under them.*

—HENRY DAVID THOREAU

Before seeking genes for a disorder using the sophisticated methods of molecular and statistical genetics, we need to justify the search with epidemiologic data. If such data show genes to play a substantial role in the etiology of the disorder, then we would likely proceed with molecular genetic studies. Otherwise, we would do better to study environmental causes.

This chapter describes the three basic tools of psychiatric genetics: family, twin, and adoption studies. As Table 2.1 shows, these studies focus on fundamental questions of psychiatric genetics: How can we be certain that a disorder runs in families? And how can we disentangle the effects of genes from those of a complex and changing environment? Later chapters will show how variations of these studies can clarify the heterogeneity of psychiatric disorders and eventually identify specific mental illness genes.

For each method we first describe the basics you need to understand its logic and illustrate how it has clarified the etiology of a mental illness. Next, we present technical details for each method. Although these tech-

TABLE 2.1. Three Basic Genetic Epidemiologic Designs

Type of study	Questions the design answers
Family study	Does the disorder run in families?
Twin study	Do genes, environmental factors, or some combination of the two cause the disorder?
Adoption study	Can the familial transmission of a disorder be attributed to genes or to the psychosocial milieu of the family?

nical sections can be skipped if all you seek at the moment are the rudiments of psychiatric genetic methodology, we hope that you will eventually read them because, as a consumer of psychiatric genetic research, knowledge of these technical tools will help you judge the quality of research reports or reviews of the literature. You do not need to be a geneticist, epidemiologist, or statistician to understand the meaning and value of psychiatric genetic research. But if you have a basic understanding of methodologic principles, you will be better able to evaluate psychiatric genetic research reports. Moreover, in some cases, the technical points of psychiatric genetics can be used in your clinical evaluation of patients or your communications to them about genetic risk.

IS A DISORDER FAMILIAL?: THE CASE–CONTROL FAMILY STUDY

The family study method is one of the most widely used tools in psychiatric genetics. This approach answers the simple question: Does a specific psychiatric illness run in families? Logically, if genes are etiologically important to a disorder, then relatives of ill individuals should be more likely to have that particular disorder than people in the population at large.

In the shorthand of genetic epidemiology, any person who has the disorder under investigation is a "case" and the case that brings the family to the attention of the study is called a "proband." So if we search clinic records for all attention-deficit/hyperactivity disorder (ADHD) patients who have relatives willing to be studied, those clinic patients would be the case probands.

Suppose we found that the prevalence of ADHD among relatives of our ADHD probands was 25 percent, which is much higher than the population prevalence of 3–10 percent. What could we conclude? We might infer that the relatives had an unusually high prevalence of ADHD and conclude that ADHD runs in families. But we would be wrong. By limiting our study only to ADHD families, we failed to rule out the possibility that some other factor accounted for the high prevalence of ADHD in relatives. For example, perhaps we used faulty diagnostic methods that would have produced high rates of ADHD in any random group of people.

To deal with such potential biases, we need to study a group of "control" probands who do not have the disorder being studied. The control group is useful because any bias that influences the measurements and diagnoses made on case families should also influence the assessments of control families. If, in our hypothetical ADHD study, our diagnostic method overestimated ADHD among relatives, the extent of overestimation should be the same for case and control families. Thus, to determine if a disorder runs in families, we need to show that it more frequently occurs among relatives of cases than among relatives of controls.

For control probands to be useful, they must be similar to the case probands on any factor that might influence the prevalence of psychiatric illness in their families. For example, some psychiatric disorders show gender differences (e.g., depression is more common in females, alcoholism more common in males), many have a higher prevalence among people from lower social classes (e.g., schizophrenia), and most show increasing rates with age. So to make clear inferences from a family study, it is essential that cases and controls do not differ on age, sex, social class, or any other attribute believed to predict the presence of the mental illness under study.

> **Key Point:** We learn very little from simply studying the relatives of patients who have the disorder of interest. We must also study a control group if we are to draw meaningful inferences.

We will illustrate the case–control study method by using data from a study of ADHD—a childhood-onset disorder of inattention, impulsivity, and hyperactivity. The study was conducted by two of the authors (MTT and SVF) and Dr. Joseph Biederman at the Massachusetts General Hospital and Harvard Medical School. Working with Dr. Biederman, we selected 140 boys with ADHD (the "cases") and 120 boys without ADHD (the "controls").

We examined these boys, their parents, and their siblings. Figure 2.1 presents some of our results. It shows that the relatives of the boys with ADHD were more likely to have ADHD than the relatives of the control boys. This was true when fathers, mothers, brothers, and sisters

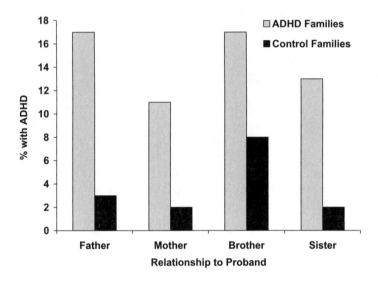

FIGURE 2.1. Family study of attention-deficit/hyperactivity disorder. Data from Faraone, S., Biederman, J., Chen, W. J., Krifcher, B., Keenan, K., Moore, C., Sprich, S., & Tsuang, M. (1992). Segregation analysis of attention deficit hyperactivity disorder: Evidence for single gene transmission. *Psychiatric Genetics*, *2*, 257–275.

were considered separately. For example, the 17 percent prevalence of ADHD in fathers of ADHD boys was significantly greater than the 3 percent prevalence in fathers of control boys. Researchers use the word "significant" as shorthand for "statistically significant," which means that, according to a statistical test, an observed difference is so large it is unlikely to be due to chance.

If we had only studied a series of ADHD children and their family members, we could have described the pattern of illness in families but we could not have determined if families of ADHD cases differed from other families. Without a control group, we might have concluded that the rates of ADHD in the ADHD families were "high" because they exceeded what others had found in epidemiologic population studies. But that conclusion would have been premature: without a control group, we could not have ruled out the possibility that our method of diagnosing ADHD was faulty. For example, if the diagnosticians had assumed that ADHD was familial, they might have rated the diagnosis as positive in ambiguous or mild cases that would not be so diagnosed in a clinic. Such "experimenter bias" effects are not necessarily intentional, but they do make it impossible to draw meaningful inferences from uncontrolled studies. In contrast, in our

ADHD study, the use of a control group made it easy to rule out faulty assessment or diagnostic procedures as the cause of our results.

Of course, a control group will not serve its purpose if the diagnosticians know which study participants are related to cases and which to controls. When this happens the assessments of family members might be biased. For example, knowing that a study subject is related to an ADHD subject might influence the assessor to make higher ratings of ADHD.

Sometimes biases are intentional. For example, diagnosticians may be so personally invested in the hypotheses of their study that they skew the data to favor their own outlook. More commonly, biased data collection will be inadvertent. How this occurs is not completely understood but that it does occur is consistent with the widely accepted premise that some human behavior is regulated, in part, by nonconscious processes. Fortunately, it is easy to eliminate both intentional and inadvertent biases: if personnel do not know who is and is not related to a case proband, then their assessments will not be influenced by assumptions related to their hypotheses. Research reports use the terms "blind" or "naive" raters to describe the individuals who assess psychopathology in family members without knowledge of the diagnosis of the proband.

In a later section we will describe the types of assessments used in family studies. Here it is worth noting that the research question will guide the choice of measures. For example, if we seek only to determine if depression is familial, then we need only assess depression among the relatives of depressed and nondepressed persons. If we are wondering if the familial risk for depression is also expressed as anxiety, then we would also assess relatives for anxiety disorders. In this manner we can use the case–control study to search for familial associations among disorders, a phenomenon that we will discuss in Chapter 3.

In the ADHD study, we examined all first-degree relatives of each proband. *First-degree relatives* are parents, siblings, or children; they share, on average, half their genes in common with the proband. Since additional genetic information can be found in more distant relatives, some studies examine *second-degree relatives*: for example, grandparents, uncles, and aunts. These relatives share, on average, one-fourth of their genes with the proband. *Third-degree relatives* (e.g., cousins) share, on average, one-eighth of their genes with the proband.

These more distant relatives are useful in family studies because, if a disorder is caused by genes, then the risk to relatives of ill probands should be related to the number of genes they share with the proband.

First-degree relatives should be at greater risk for the disorder than second-degree relatives, and second-degree relatives should be at greater risk than third-degree relatives. Thus, the idea that genes are involved in a disorder predicts that the risk to relatives of ill probands decreases as we move from close to distant relatives.

As an example, consider Figure 2.2, which summarizes several studies of the lifetime prevalence of schizophrenia among groups with different degrees of genetic relationship to a schizophrenic proband. At the top of the figure, we find the lowest risk among the general population: people who are not selected for being genetically related to a schizophrenic patient have a 1 percent prevalence of the disorder. Moving down the figure, we see a slightly higher prevalence, about 3 percent, among half-siblings, grandchildren, nephews, nieces, uncles, and aunts. These second-degree relatives share 25 percent of their genes with schizophrenic patients.

As expected from a genetic theory of schizophrenia, the first-degree relatives (siblings, children, and parents) have an even greater prevalence of the disorder, about 10 percent. Note that parents of probands have a lower risk for schizophrenia than do children of probands. Any model of genetic transmission would predict these two risks to be equal. This anomaly in the genetic prediction occurs because schizophrenia impairs a person's ability to marry and have children. Thus, schizophrenia is less frequently observed among people who have attained parenthood than those who have not.

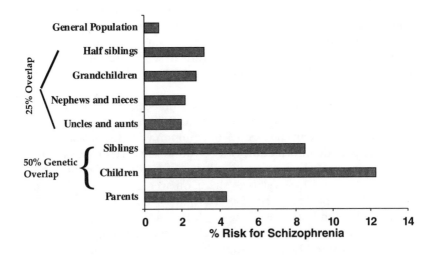

FIGURE 2.2. Lifetime prevalence of schizophrenia by degree of genetic relationship to a schizophrenic patient.

Figure 2.2 clearly shows a pattern of illness that is consistent with the idea that genes increase the risk for schizophrenia. Second-degree relatives have a higher prevalence than the general population, and the risk to first-degree relatives exceeds the risk to second-degree relatives. Although these data support the idea that genes cause schizophrenia, they are far from definitive because a disorder can be familial for other reasons. For example, family members share a common culture and a common environment. The similarity of these factors tends to increase as the degree of relationship decreases.

Thus, familial environmental factors may affect genetic relationships in ways not readily apparent. For example, if cigarette smoking is a habit that children learn from parents, then one might observe that smoking-related disorders such as emphysema run in families. Yet the familial transmission of such a disorder may be due entirely to relatives sharing a common environmental pathogen. Possible sources of cultural and environmental transmission include bacteria, viruses, learned responses to stress, and cultural differences in emotional expression. Since a disorder can run in a family for nongenetic reasons, the finding of familial transmission cannot be unambiguously interpreted as genetic in origin.

> **Key Point:** Showing that a disorder runs in families does not conclusively establish that genes cause the disorder. Although family studies are indispensable for establishing the familial transmission of disorders, they cannot by themselves establish the causes of those disorders. All mechanisms that could lead to a familial clustering of disease should be considered. To disentangle genetic and environmental causes of familial transmission, we must use either a twin study or an adoption study.

Evaluating Family Studies

When evaluating a family study, you should attend to two key questions: How were the families selected? How were the family members evaluated?

How Were the Families Selected?

As mentioned earlier in this chapter, a family study should use the blind case–control paradigm, a staple of epidemiology and behavioral science. The cases and controls used in genetic studies are called "probands." We can either select probands directly from the general population or we can use a source, such as a psychiatric clinic or hospital, that is likely to have many potential probands with the disorder of interest. Population-based and clinic-based studies have different strengths and weaknesses that we need to consider in either planning or evaluating a family study.

The major strength of a population-based family study is that it allows us to generalize results from the specific sample studied to the entire population. In contrast, the probands from clinic-based studies may not be representative of the full range of the disorder as it occurs in the population. From epidemiologic studies we know that many cases of mental illness are not referred for treatment and that there are systematic differences between referred and nonreferred cases. The most notable difference is that referred cases are more likely to have multiple mental disorders than nonreferred ones.

Yet epidemiologic-based family studies face several practical problems. Although it is theoretically possible to create a sample that is representative of the population, in practice this ideal is difficult to achieve. For example, some population-based studies sample through the telephone directory, thus missing potential subjects who do not have telephones. Others sample children through public schools, thereby missing potential subjects who attend private schools or who are placed in long-term residential care settings.

We should also consider that although a clinic-based study may not be representative of the entire population of cases, it will be relevant to clinically referred cases. Since such cases are of most interest to clinicians, studying them to the exclusion of others is not much of a liability.

> **Key Point:** Findings from studies that select participants from the community may not apply to patients selected from clinics. The converse is also true: findings from studies that select patients from clinics may not apply to cases of illness found in the community.

But the major advantage of clinic-based studies is that they are easier and less expensive to implement than population-based epidemiologic studies. For example, consider the expense of screening the general population for probands with schizophrenia, which has a population prevalence of about 1 percent. To find 100 probands we would need to screen 10,000 people. In contrast, it is relatively easy to find 100 schizophrenic probands in clinical settings that care for these patients.

In addition to creating a practical problem, the low prevalence of disorders in the general population has an adverse effect on the accuracy of the diagnoses made in the study. This occurs because we can never be 100 percent sure that a diagnosis is correct. Diagnostic inaccuracy comes from many sources, including lack of information, fluctuations in the patient's clinical state over time, errors of clinical inference, and errors in coding diagnoses. We can summarize the implications of these errors in two statistics: (1) the *sensitivity of a diagnosis* is the probability that we correctly diagnose an ill person as ill, and (2) the *false-positive rate* is the probability that we incorrectly diagnose a well person as ill.

Now consider this example. Suppose that our diagnosis of schizophrenia has a diagnostic sensitivity of 90 percent and a false-positive rate of only 1 percent. These figures mean that we will correctly diagnose 90 out of 100 schizophrenics but will misdiagnose 1 out of 100 nonschizophrenics as schizophrenic. In a sample of 10,000 people, 100 will have schizophrenia and 9,900 will not. Thus, our diagnostic procedure will find 90 schizophrenics among the 100 true schizophrenics but it will also diagnose 1 percent or 99 of the 9,900 nonschizophrenics as ill. In total we will diagnose 189 people with schizophrenia but more than 52 percent will not have schizophrenia.

In contrast, consider what happens when we select cases from a mental health center that treats 500 outpatients, 400 of whom are schizophrenic. Our diagnostic procedure will diagnose as schizophrenic 360 of the 400 schizophrenics and only 1 of the nonschizophrenics. Thus, our false positive rate will be less than 1 percent, much less than the 52 percent false-positive rate from the epidemiologic study.

> **Key Point:** Studies that select patients from clinics make fewer false-positive diagnostic errors than studies that select patients from the community.

These statistical considerations motivate a methodological maxim: *when our goal is to minimize the false-positive rate of diagnosis, it is essential that we select subjects from a source that has a high prevalence of the disorder.* Mental health clinics and hospitals are the obvious choice for finding groups of people with high rates of mental illness.

Just as cases should come from a source that has a high prevalence of the disorder, so should controls come from a source that has a high prevalence of people not having the disorder. For example, if we select controls from a general medical clinic, we will be assured that the underlying prevalence of schizophrenia in the source of controls will be low so that our diagnoses of "not schizophrenic" will mostly be correct.

We emphasize that controls should be screened only for the disorder being studied, not for other psychiatric disorders or conditions. When controls are screened for additional disorders, the results can spuriously indicate a familial relationship between the disorder used to select cases and the disorders that were screened from controls. For example, we know that BOTH alcoholism and anxiety disorders run in families. Consider a family study that uses controls who have neither alcoholism nor anxiety disorders and compares these with alcoholic patients. Since anxiety disorders run in families, the prevalence of anxiety among relatives of controls will be decreased by the method of selection. In contrast, the rates in relatives of alcoholics will not be decreased. Thus, anxiety disorders will be more prevalent among the relatives of alcoholics due to the choice of control group.

> **Key Point:** The control group should be comparable to the patient group on all other factors except the presence of disease.

The selection of controls should satisfy the comparability principles required for meaningful inferences in case–control epidemiological studies. Ideally, we would like our controls to be people who would have been cases had they developed the disorder of interest during the time of investigation. When sampling cases from a mental health clinic, this requires that if the control subjects had needed treatment for the disorder, they probably would have been referred to the same mental health clinic that provided the case probands. For example, in a general hospital outpatient setting, it is likely that patients who seek treatment for medical disorders in medical clinics would go to the same hospital's psychiatric clinic for the treatment of a psychiatric disorder.

One way to assure that cases and controls will be comparable is to choose controls who are "matched" to the cases on variables that are associated with the presence or absence of the mental illness to be studied. For example, schizophrenia is more common among lower social classes, depression is more common among women than men and most psychiatric disorders show an increasing prevalence with age. If cases and controls differ on any of these key variables, it will be difficult to draw meaningful inferences.

If our schizophrenic probands came from low social strata but our controls came from high social strata, then a finding of higher rates of schizophrenia among relatives of schizophrenic probands would not be interpretable. Thus, schizophrenic and control probands should be "matched" on social class. We could either use *group matching*, which requires that the mean social class level is the same for the schizophrenic and control groups, or *explicit matching*, which requires that for each schizophrenic proband we have a control proband from the same social stratum.

Matching, however, should be used cautiously so as to avoid "overmatching." Thus, matching on specific variables often unmatches on others. An obvious example of overmatching is as follows. Numerous studies find that ADHD interferes with school achievement. Thus, matching ADHD subjects to controls on school achievement would create an unusually high functioning ADHD sample or an unusually low functioning control sample. It would be difficult to draw meaningful inferences from comparing such samples.

Following the selection of cases and controls, the study attempts to assess the diagnostic status of as many of the relatives of cases and controls as possible. The aim is to compare rates of illness in relatives of cases to rates of illness in the relatives of controls. To accurately estimate these rates of illness care must be taken to assess as many relatives as possible. Yet, because psychiatric disorders affect emotions, thinking and interpersonal relationships, nonparticipation may not be random with respect to illness status: family members who are ill are more likely to refuse participation than those who are well. Paranoid schizophrenia provides a good example of this problem. Paranoia leads to distrusts of strangers, friends, and family. This makes it difficult for a paranoid person to agree to answer the many questions required by psychiatric interviews. To avoid such problems, high participation rates are needed. In practice, this can be difficult, but it can be achieved by using a clinically sensitive approach at a time when the subject's illness is less likely to interfere with his or her participation.

How Were Family Members Evaluated?

In this section we focus on the implications for research of the methods used to assess family members. But in addition to its implications for the design and evaluation of research, this section is also directly relevant to the clinical task of taking a family history—a topic which we discuss at length in Chapter 6.

Family studies of psychiatric illness choose between two ways of evaluating family members: the family history and the family study methods. The family history method collects diagnostic information about family members by interviewing only one or several informants per family. This method uses a specialized interview form such as Dr.

Nancy Andreasen's Family History Research Diagnostic Criteria (FH-RDC) interview or the National Institute of Mental Health (NIMH) Genetics Initiative's Family Interview for Genetic Studies (FIGS).

In contrast, the family study method determines diagnoses by interviewing all family members in person. Several excellent structured psychiatric interviews are available but only one was designed specifically for genetic studies: the NIMH Genetics Initiative's Diagnostic Interview for Genetic Studies.

An obvious advantage of the family history method is its low cost: interviewing one family member about the entire family is less costly than interviewing all the family members. Thus, in clinical practice one frequently takes a family history from the patient or a close relative but rarely interviews many of the patient's relatives in person.

Family history data, however, underestimate the true prevalence of many psychiatric disorders. We know this to be true because several studies have collected family history data on the same subjects who have also been diagnosed by the family study method. By using the family study method as the "gold standard," researchers have estimated the accuracy of the family history method and shown it to be wanting. Taken together, these studies show that the family history method fails to correctly diagnose many family members who are truly ill. But because it rarely diagnoses a well person as ill, we still consider it to be a useful method.

> **Key Point:** Information collected by directly interviewing a family member is much more accurate than information collected from informants concerning that family member.

The low accuracy of the family history method does not compromise the results of a case–control study, but it does make it more difficult to find evidence for familial transmission. Additionally, when reading the results of a family history paper, one must remember that the risk to relatives it presents is an underestimate. In clinical settings, the family history method is useful, but clinicians should be alert to the fact that, although a positive diagnosis is probably correct, the lack of one has a high probability of being wrong.

Fortunately, it is possible to improve the accuracy of the family history method by using five procedures that have been validated in the research literature (Table 2.2). Given the waxing and waning nature of many psychiatric symptoms, it is very important that you have at least one informant who has had substantial contact with the subject being

TABLE 2.2. Procedures to Improve the Family History Method

1. Use informants who have had substantial contact with the subject.

2. Use multiple informants.

3. Remember that a diagnosis is more likely to be accurate if the *subject* is currently ill but less likely to be accurate if the *informant* is ill.

4. Use a semistructured interview.

5. Use less stringent diagnostic criteria

diagnosed. Someone who has lived with the subject for some time is ideal. If possible, use multiple informants and conclude that the subject has the disorder if any of the informants provide data to that effect.

You can also improve the accuracy of your family history diagnoses by remembering that a positive diagnosis is more likely to be correct if the relative being diagnosed is ill at the time of the family history interview. This makes intuitive sense: we are more likely to know of a relative's problems if, for example, he or she is in a psychiatric hospital at the time we ask about the individual's condition.

You must also consider the possibility that informants may be less accurate if they themselves are psychiatrically ill. In some cases this is obvious from the patient's clinical state: the actively psychotic schizophrenic or the agitated depressive cannot be expected to provide much valid information. But the validity of informant reports is also suspect if they have *ever* had a disorder. Dr. Kenneth Kendler and colleagues showed this by asking discordant twins about depression, anxiety, and alcoholism in their parents. Twins are discordant if only one has the disease being studied. Compared with the unaffected twin, those twins with a history of major depression or generalized anxiety were more likely to report the same disorder in their parents. Note, however, that this effect was not observed for alcoholism.

If you use one of the semistructured interviews developed for taking family histories, you will more efficiently assess each of the signs and symptoms relevant to the disorder. That, in turn, will lead to more accurate diagnoses. Moreover, when you make a diagnosis using family history data, you should use a less stringent decision rule than you would if you had completed an in-person interview. Table 2.3 shows examples of the schizophrenia and depression rules from Dr. Andreasen's FH-RDC instrument. If you compare these rules with those from DSM-IV or other diagnostic systems, you will see that the FH-RDC requires fewer signs and symptoms than do the corresponding DSM-IV diagnoses.

TABLE 2.3. Examples of Less Stringent Diagnostic Criteria

Family History Criteria for Schizophrenia (A, B, and C are required)

A. No prominent symptoms of a mood disturbance

B. At least one of the following:
   1. Delusions
   2. Hallucinations
   3. Incoherence
   4. Grossly bizarre behavior

C. Evidence of an illness that lasted at least one year without recovery

Family History Criteria for Depression (A through E are required)

A. Evidence of a dysphoric mood change to either:
   1. A depressive mood
   2. Another dysphoric mood (e.g., anxious, irritable) plus two of the following: Loss of interest, appetite or weight change, sleep change, loss of energy, psychomotor agitation or retardation, guilt or self-reproach, impaired concentration

B. At least one of the following is associated with the symptoms in A: Electroconvulsive therapy, antidepressant medication, hospitalization, suicidal behavior, treatment for dysphoric mood change, gross functional impairment, four of the symptoms listed in A2

C. No evidence suggestive of a chronic, nonaffective deterioration

D. No evidence that the period lasted less than two weeks

E. Does not meet criteria for schizoaffective disorder

Note. Data from Andreasen, N. C., Endicott, J., Spitzer, R. L., & Winokur, G. (1977). The family history method using diagnostic criteria: Reliability and validity. *Archives of General Psychiatry, 34,* 1229–1235.

For example, the DSM-IV diagnosis of depression requires that a dysphoric mood change last for at least two weeks; the FH-RDC diagnosis has no duration requirement. The DSM-IV diagnosis requires the presence of four depressive symptoms in addition to the mood change; the FH-RDC requires only one or two depending on the nature of the mood change. The use of less stringent diagnoses makes it easier for subjects to be diagnosed. Thus, more subjects will be diagnosed than would have been diagnosed if the full criteria were used. Research suggests that the use of these less stringent diagnoses improves the family history method of detecting true cases without markedly increasing the number of well family members incorrectly diagnosed as ill.

> **Clinical Tip:** In clinical practice, the forms created for assessing family history (the FH-RDC and the FIGS) are useful tools for systematically collecting psychiatric information about the relatives of your patients.

TABLE 2.4. Family Study vs. Family History Method

Method	Advantages	Disadvantages
Family history	Practical Few false-positive diagnoses	Many false-negative diagnoses
Family study	Few false-positive or false-negative diagnoses	Expensive

Ideally, the diagnoses of subjects should use three sources of information: direct interviews with the subject, family history interviews with informants who are familiar with the subject, and medical records when available. All sources of information are then combined into a consensus diagnosis according to the judgment of an experienced clinician. Several studies have shown that the direct interview and medical record usually provide more useful information than the family history assessment. In fact, diagnoses based on direct interviews alone closely approximate best estimate diagnoses. A diagnosis based only on medical records, however, is often a suitable proxy for the best estimate diagnosis.

Table 2.4 outlines the advantages and disadvantages of the family history and family study methods. The choice between the two requires a trade-off between data quality and the expense of data collection. The family history method is the method of choice when there are not sufficient data to justify the expense of a family study. Thus, it is a good choice for pilot phases of a genetic investigation. However, after the family history method demonstrates familiality, the family study is the tool of choice for precisely estimating the degree of familial transmission.

IS THE DISORDER GENETIC?: TWIN STUDIES

The occurrence of twinning provides a powerful, natural experiment in human genetics. Monozygotic (MZ) or identical twins share 100 percent of their genes with each other. Thus, differences between MZ twins must be due to environmental influences. Dizygotic (DZ) or fraternal twins share only 50 percent of their genes with one another; their genetic similarity is the same as that between siblings. DZ twins are not genetic copies of one another but like MZ twins they share a common environment from birth. Thus, if genes cause a disorder, then the MZ co-twins of ill probands should be at higher risk for the disorder than the DZ co-twins of ill probands.

> **Key Point:** If genes predispose to a disorder, then it should co-occur more among MZ twins than among DZ twins.

You can appreciate the power of the twin method immediately by considering this simple fact: the prevalence of schizophrenia among MZ co-twins of schizophrenic probands is about 55 percent, which is much greater than the 10 percent risk to same-sex DZ twins. These schizophrenia twin data are remarkable for two reasons. First, they unequivocally show that genes play a role in causing schizophrenia. Indeed, having a schizophrenic MZ co-twin is the most robust predictor of schizophrenia known to science.

Second, and equally remarkable, is what these twin data indicate about schizophrenia and the environment: the studies of MZ twins tell us that nearly half of all people who have a schizophrenic co-twin will not become schizophrenic themselves. Why would only one of a pair of genetically identical persons have schizophrenia? Only one answer is possible: some environmental feature must have triggered schizophrenia in the ill co-twin.

Do the schizophrenia twin data mean that half the causes of schizophrenia are genetic and half environmental? Or are half of schizophrenic cases caused by genes and half by adverse environments? The answer is a bit more complicated than these questions presume. It lies in a careful understanding of how geneticists use mathematical methods to quantify the relative role of genes and environment. Although the following paragraphs are somewhat technical, they are worth making the effort to read carefully because the questions they answer are among the most frequent that psychiatric patients and their families have when discussing the role of genes in mental illness.

> **Clinical Tip:** We use the word "vulnerability" as shorthand for the aggregate of genetic and environmental risk factors that determine risk for developing a disease. Like weight, vulnerability comes in all sizes, with the larger sizes creating the greatest risks for illness. Think of interventions, be they pharmacologic or psychosocial, as reducing vulnerability. The concept of vulnerability and its implications for understanding the effects of treatment can be useful tools for explaining to patients how therapies work in the context of their disease.

We will first take a short detour and discuss in more detail the concept of "vulnerability" introduced in Chapter 1. This term refers to an individual's unobservable predisposition to develop a disorder. As you will recall from the first chapter's discussion of complex inheritance (see Figure 1.1), each of us can, theoretically, be described as being exposed to a set of genes and environmental insults that determine our susceptibility to developing a psychiatric disorder. This vulnerability cannot be directly measured, so we can only describe it using hypothetical data, as in Figure 2.3.

As Figure 2.3 indicates, unlike psychiatric diagnoses, vulnerability is not a binary category. Instead, it is a quantitative trait (like physical traits such as height or psychological traits such as intelligence) that varies from very low levels to very high levels. Most people have moderate levels of vulnerability; fewer people have very high or very low levels. When a person's vulnerability exceeds the threshold denoted T in the figure he or she will be affected by the psychiatric disorder associated with the unobservable vulnerability. We call Figure 2.3 a "multifactorial" vulnerability model because it assumes that many genes and environmental effects combine to create an individual's susceptibility to becoming ill.

One reason for considering the multifactorial model is that we know it is accurate for some disorders for which vulnerability can be directly measured. For example, some heart attacks occur when the amount of cholesterol in the blood gets so high as to clog blood vessels and interfere with cardiac functioning. In this case, the underlying but measurable vulnerability is the cholesterol level. When this exceeds a specific threshold (the point at which arteries are clogged), a heart attack ensues.

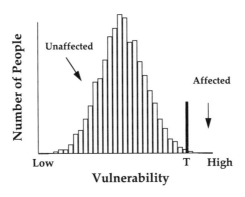

FIGURE 2.3. Multifactorial model of vulnerability.

Partitioning Genetic and Environmental Sources of Illness

As Figure 2.3 shows, the level of vulnerability varies from person to person. The mathematical geneticist attempts to explain this variability by using twin data. The basic idea is to partition the causes of disorders into the three sources given in Table 2.5: heritability, common environment, and unique environment. *Heritability* measures the degree to which the vulnerability to develop a disorder is influenced by genes. A value of 0 indicates that vulnerability is due entirely to environmental influences; a value of 1 indicates that the liability can be explained entirely by genes; intermediate values express the proportion of liability that is due to genes.

As Table 2.5 indicates, there are two environmental causes: common environment and unique environment. *Common or shared environment* refers to environmental factors shared by twins. Examples of shared environment are social class and exposure to parental conflict. The presence of shared environmental risk factors for a disorder will make twins more similar to one another than would be expected from the amount of genes they have in common.

Unique environment assesses the portion of vulnerability due to environmental factors not shared by twins. Examples of nonshared sources of environment are exposure to peer groups and number and type of birth complications. Unique environmental factors will make twins less similar to one another.

The methods for computing the genetic and environmental sources of variability are beyond the scope of this book. Instead, we will turn next to examples of how these methods have been used to clarify the genetic and environmental causes of psychiatric disorders. Our first example comes from a review of European twin studies of manic–depressive psychosis. For each study, Figure 2.4 shows the portion of manic–depressive etiology that can be attributed to genes, common environment, and unique environment. Notably, most of these studies agree that genes account for the largest portion of the etiology of the

TABLE 2.5. Disentangling Genes from Environment in Twin Studies

Source of variance	Definition
Heritability	Portion of vulnerability due to genes
Common environment	Portion of vulnerability due to environmental factors shared by twins
Unique environment	Portion of vulnerability due to environmental factors not shared by twins

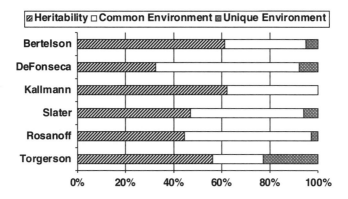

FIGURE 2.4. Sources of variance from twin studies of mood disorders. Data from Tsuang, M. T., & Faraone, S. V. (1990). *The genetics of mood disorders.* Baltimore: Johns Hopkins University Press.

disorder. But they also show that the effects of the shared environment cannot be ignored. In contrast, unique environmental risk factors appear to play a small role in the etiology of manic–depressive psychosis.

> **Key Point:** Although twin studies are often branded as "genetic" research, they tell us as much about the environment as they do about genes. In fact, twin studies provide the most solid evidence for what clinicians have known for years: the environment plays a substantial role in causing most types of mental illness.

We will illustrate a more complex use of the twin method by employing data from a twin study of antisocial personality. This study was conducted by Dr. Michael Lyons from Boston University, two of the authors (MTT and SVF) at Harvard Medical School, and colleagues from Washington University and the Hines Department of Veterans Affairs (VA) Medical Center. It assessed juvenile and adult antisocial traits among 1,788 MZ and 1,438 DZ pairs of adult male twins from the VA's Vietnam Era Twin Registry.

Figure 2.5 gives results from the mathematical genetic analysis of these twin data. The figure presents two pie charts, one for juvenile antisocial traits and one for adult antisocial traits. The juvenile chart shows that most of the variability in juvenile antisocial behavior could be attributed to environmental causes—the heritability was nearly zero. In contrast, for adult antisocial traits, the heritability estimate indicated

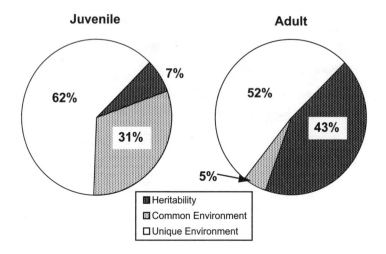

FIGURE 2.5. Effects of genes and environment on antisocial traits. Data from Lyons, M. J., True, W. R., Eisen, S. A., Goldberg, J., Meyer, J. M., Faraone, S. V., Eaves, L. J., & Tsuang, M. T. (1995). Differential heritability of adult and juvenile antisocial traits. *Archives of General Psychiatry, 52,* 906–915.

that 43 percent of adult antisocial behavior could be attributed to genes. Thus, the effect of genes on antisocial behavior was stronger in adulthood than in childhood.

Of course, this changing heritability with age means that the impact of the environment also must change with development. As Figure 2.5 shows, juvenile antisocial traits were almost entirely explained by common and unique environmental factors, with the latter having twice the effect of the former. In contrast, common environmental factors did not influence the expression of adult antisocial traits but unique environmental factors accounted for about half their variability.

These results make good clinical sense. As juveniles, twins share more of a common environment than they do as adults. In their youth they live in the same home, play in the same neighborhood, and attend the same schools. As adults, these and other aspects of the common environment attenuate, leaving more of a role to be played by genes and unique environment.

Of course, because we did not measure specific aspects of the environment, our comments about which environmental features change over time are hypotheses, not facts. This highlights a weakness of the twin method when the researcher only collects data about psychiatric disorders: it can tell us that the environment plays a causal role in these disorders, but it cannot tell us the nature of these environmental causes unless explicit measures of the environment are added to the study design.

Our twin study of antisocial personality highlights a crucial issue in the interpretation of heritability: *the effects of genes on a disorder can change through the life cycle.* At first blush this might seem odd to you. After all, we are born with our entire set of genes and retain these through adulthood. Shouldn't their effects on behavior be static over time? The answer is no. When you understand why, you will have a fuller comprehension of the concept of heritability.

Consider the following simplified situation: a twin study of disease X in 1995 shows it to have a heritability of 100 percent. This means that genes are the only cause of the disorder. This could either occur if no aspect of the environment could facilitate or stop the emergence of disease X. It could also occur if such an environmental factor did exist, but none of the twins who were studied had been exposed to that factor. Now suppose we conducted another twin study in a region of the country where twins had been exposed to a feature of the environment that could stop the progression of disease X. That study would compute a heritability of, for example, 60 percent.

So, which study is correct? Does the disorder have a heritability of 100 percent or of 60 percent? Actually, both studies should be considered to be correct; however, we must remember that their results cannot be generalized to people exposed to different environments. The key point we wish to make here is that any estimate of heritability depends on what sample is being studied, what genes occur in the sample, and the nature of the environment to which members of the sample have been exposed.

In our antisocial twin study it is possible that the effects of genes stayed the same from juvenile to adult years but exposure to environmental factors diminished. That would lead to an increase in the computed heritability from juvenile to adult years. It is also conceivable that the increased heritability in adult years was caused by changes in the genetic contribution to etiology. This would occur if genes relevant to antisocial traits were turned on or off during development. For example, the human brain is not fully developed until early adulthood, with the neural connections to the frontal lobes being among the last to be formed. So, if the effects of a specific gene are mediated through the frontal lobes, then that source of genetic etiology would not take effect until late adolescence or early adulthood.

Thus, we conclude that any estimate of the relative importance of genes and environment should be interpreted cautiously. Such estimates are not immutable facts of nature. They are snapshots of the changing landscape created by the confluence of genes and environment.

> **Key Point:** Heritability is a useful index of the relative importance of genes and environment in causing a disease. But high heritabilities do not mean that patients are fated to endure the inexorable effects of pathogenic genes. By changing the biologic, psychologic, or social environment, effective treatments can reduce heritability as they mitigate, cure, and eventually prevent disease.

The fact that heritability may change with development has implications for how clinicians communicate psychiatric genetic information to patients and their families. This idea keeps open the possibility that modifications to the environment might lessen their genetic risks for the disorder. For example, from a mathematical perspective, preventive interventions seek to increase the amount of environmental variance in families. If this variance is therapeutic, it will reduce the likelihood of disease expression and diminish the heritability of the disorder.

A convenient way to describe for patients the interplay of genes and environment is to use a simple example: retardation due to phenylketonuria (PKU). Infants who inherit two aberrant PKU genes have a complete deficiency of the enzyme required to metabolize phenylalanine. The resulting high levels of phenylalanine are toxic to the brain and lead to mental retardation. But these children will become retarded *only* if they ingest phenylalanine. So, on the one hand, PKU seems to be a "genetic" disorder because of the mutant gene that prevents adequate phenylalanine metabolism. On the other hand, PKU seems to be an "environmental" condition because one must ingest phenylalanine to become ill.

In most human environments, everyone ingests phenylalanine because it is a common constituent of protein-containing foods. Thus, there are no relevant environmental differences among people (i.e., everyone ingests enough phenylalanine to become sick if they have the mutant genes). In contrast, there are genetic differences: only some people carry the two copies of the mutated gene that leads to PKU. Thus, the heritability of PKU under normal environmental conditions is 100 percent.

Now let us do a thought experiment. Imagine a world where all humans carried the two PKU genes but only some ingested phenylalanine. In this situation, there would be no relevant genetic variability but some environmental variability. Heritability would be zero and we would view PKU as an "environmental" disorder due to the toxin phenylalanine.

Evaluating Twin Studies

The ability of the twin method to provide meaningful results is inextricably linked with its ability to correctly determine zygosity, that is, whether a pair of twins is MZ or DZ. A substantial misclassification of MZ twins as DZ or vice versa would lead to meaningless results. Fortunately, precise methods of zygosity determination exist: laboratory analysis can precisely characterize small stretches of our genetic material, DNA.

Because the DNA of MZ twins must be identical, a twin-pair can be classified as DZ if the twins differ on any stretch of DNA. Many pieces of DNA have been described, so it is possible to make the probability of misclassification very low. In the absence of DNA data, similarity of physical characteristics such as eye color and dermatoglyphics can provide accurate estimates of zygosity. In fact, determination of zygosity by response to questions about the degree of physical similarity and the degree to which the twins were mistaken for one another as children has been shown to be reasonably accurate in comparison to genetic marker classifications. Although zygosity can theoretically be determined with high accuracy, even sophisticated methods using genetic markers are subject to experimental and laboratory error. Thus, some confusion between MZ and DZ twins is to be expected although it appears unlikely that zygosity errors will greatly influence results if appropriate procedures are followed.

Inferences from twin studies to non-twin populations may be inappropriate if biologic or psychosocial factors associated with twinning are etiologically important in the development of psychiatric disorders. For example, compared with non-twins, twins have lower birth weights, suffer from higher rates of pregnancy and delivery complications, and are more likely to have congenital malformations. Since pregnancy and delivery complications can have neurologic sequelae relevant to the etiology of psychiatric disorders, these environmental influences may play a greater role in twin than in non-twin populations. For example, one study found that twins were more likely to show evidence of minimal brain dysfunction compared with a matched non-twin group. Thus, because there may be systematic differences between twins and non-twins, estimates of heritability from twin studies may not generalize to non-twins.

To examine this issue further, psychiatric geneticists have compared the psychiatric histories of twins and non-twins. For example, in a Norwegian study, Dr. Einar Kringlen tabulated the rates of first admissions for psychosis for twins and the general population. This work showed that twins were neither more nor less likely to develop schizophrenia, manic–depressive disorder, or reactive psychosis than people from the general population. Since other studies have reported similar results, it seems reasonable to assume that, for psychiatric studies, the twin method is not compromised by systematic differences between twins and non-twins.

The validity of twin studies also requires us to assume that differences between MZ and DZ twins are due to genes; we must assume that the environmental determinants of similarity are identical for the two types of twin-pairs. But if the similarity of MZ twin environments is greater than that of DZ twin environments, then the twin method will overestimate the importance of genetic influences.

The possibility of greater environmental similarity for MZ twins cannot be ignored. Several studies have found that the social environments of MZ twins are more similar than those of DZ twins. For example, habits, activities, personal preferences, parental treatment, and self-image tend to be more similar between MZ twins. Moreover, MZ twins are more likely to be dressed alike and are more likely to be confused for one another in childhood. Thus, twin studies may overestimate heritability if these differences in environmental similarity are etiologically relevant to the disorder under study.

On the other hand, the greater physical and environmental similarity of MZ twins may actually lead to a decrease in behavioral similarity. MZ twins may work harder to develop a persona that clearly differentiates each from the other. Such effects may lead to "role differentiation" where each twin performs different behavioral functions for the twin-pair (e.g., one twin may be dominant, the other submissive). Supportive of this finding is the idea that MZ twins reared apart are more similar in personality than those reared together.

For studies of psychiatric disorders, users of the twin method must be alert to the possibility of *assortative mating*, the tendency for patients with a disorder to marry a spouse who also has the disorder. Assortative mating among parents will make their DZ twin children more genetically similar to one another than expected when there is no assortative mating. This occurs because when spouses have the same genetic disorder, they are more genetically alike than spouses who do not have the same genetic disorder. Since MZ twins are always genetically identical, assortative mating has no effect on their genetic similarity. Thus, the presence of assortative mating will increase DZ similarity, leading to an underestimate of heritability.

> **Key Point:** Although some methodologic problems limit the effectiveness of twin studies, there is no conclusive evidence that these limitations substantially bias twin study results. Instead, there is a consensus among psychiatric geneticists that the twin method provides an informative source of converging evidence in determining the importance of genetic factors in psychiatric disorders.

IS THE DISORDER GENETIC?: ADOPTION STUDIES

Adoption studies provide another method of disentangling genetic and environmental contributions to the familial aggregation of a disorder. This is so because children adopted at an early age have a primarily genetic relationship with their biological parents and a totally environmental relationship with their adoptive parents. If genes are responsible for the familial transmission of a disorder, we should observe transmission from parents to natural children but not from parents to adopted children. As described in Table 2.6, there are four types of adoption study: the parent as proband study, the adoptee as proband study, the cross-fostering study, and the paternal half-sibling study.

The parent as proband study uses ill and well parents as probands and examines the prevalence of disorders among their offspring who had been adopted into other families. If genes cause the disorder being studied, then illness should be more common among the adopted-away children of ill parents than the adopted-away children of well parents.

In the first psychiatric adoption study, Dr. Leonard Heston used the parent as proband design. He examined 47 children who had been separated from their biological schizophrenic mothers within three

TABLE 2.6. Types of Adoption Studies

Type of study	Groups compared
Parent as proband	Adopted-away offspring of ill and well parents
Adoptee as proband	Biologic and adoptive relatives of ill and well adoptees
Cross-fostering	Children having ill biological parents raised by well adoptive parents and those with well biological parents raised by ill adoptive parents.
Paternal half-sibling	Biologic paternal half-siblings of ill and well adoptees

days of birth. These children were raised by adoptive parents with whom they had no biological relationship. He also examined a control group of 50 persons who had been separated from nonschizophrenic mothers. Both groups studied were adults at the time of examination.

If genes caused schizophrenia, then the biologic children of schizophrenic mothers should have a higher risk for schizophrenia regardless of who raised them as children. In contrast, if the parenting relationship—an environmental factor—caused schizophrenia, then separating children from a schizophrenic parent should prevent them from having schizophrenia. Dr. Heston's results supported a genetic etiology for schizophrenia: five children of schizophrenic mothers became schizophrenic; in contrast, none of the children of nonschizophrenic mothers became schizophrenic.

The adoptee as proband study uses ill and well adoptees as probands and assesses the prevalence of disorder in the biologic and adoptive relatives of these probands. This study concludes that genes are operative if (1) the biologic relatives of ill adoptees are at greater risk for illness than the adoptive relatives of ill adoptees and (2) the biologic parents of ill adoptees show a greater prevalence of the disorder than the biologic parents of the well adoptees.

Astudy of bipolar disorder by Drs. Julien Mendlewicz and John Rainer provides an excellent example of the adoptee as proband study. They supplemented the adoptee as proband design with two additional control groups, the parents of nonadoptees with bipolar disorder and the parents of individuals who had contracted poliomyelitis during childhood or adolescence. The purpose of the latter group was to control for the effect on parents of raising a disabled child.

As Figure 2.6 shows, Drs. Mendlewicz and Rainer found more mood disorders among the biologic in comparison with the adoptive parents of bipolar adoptees or the parents of normal adoptees. Overall, the results of Drs. Mendlewicz and Rainer's adoption study indicate that genetic, not environmental, factors are implicated in the familial transmission of bipolar disorder.

The cross-fostering study compares two group of adoptees. One group has ill biological parents but is raised by well adoptive parents. The other has well biological parents but is raised by ill adoptive parents. This design allows for a direct comparison of environmental and biological transmission in an adoptee sample.

Dr. Seymour Kety and colleagues conducted an adoption study in Denmark that included (1) adoptees who had been born of nonschizophrenic parents but raised by a schizophrenic parent and 2) adoptees who had been born to schizophrenic parents but raised by nonschizophrenic parents. According to the logic of the cross-fostering study, if

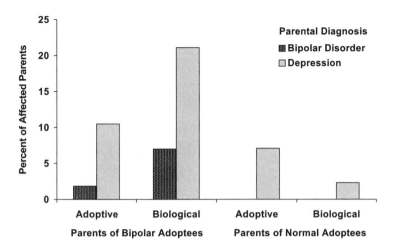

FIGURE 2.6. Bipolar disorder and depression among the adoptive and biologic parents of bipolar and normal adoptees. Data from Mendlewicz, J., & Rainer, J. D. (1977). Adoption study supporting genetic transmission in manic–depressive illness. *Nature, 268,* 327–329.

rearing by a schizophrenic parent caused schizophrenia, then the first group should be at higher risk for schizophrenia. This was not the case. Because the second group had a higher prevalence of schizophrenia, the investigators concluded that rearing by a schizophrenic parent was not a significant cause of schizophrenia.

The paternal half-sibling study was invented to solve an inferential problem faced by adoption studies: even if children were adopted-away at birth, they still would have had some contact with their mother both *in utero* and immediately after birth. It is conceivable that such experiences could influence the transmission of psychiatric illness from mother to child.

To address this problem for their adoption study of schizophrenia, Dr. Kety and his colleagues identified a group of adoptees who had paternal half-siblings, that is, siblings who shared the same biological father but a different biological mother. Because paternal half-siblings do not share pre-, peri-, or neonatal environmental exposure to the same mother, examining paternal half-siblings rules out confounding by *in utero* influences, birth traumas, and early mothering experience. In Dr. Kety's work, the biologic paternal half-siblings of schizophrenic adoptees were at greater risk for schizophrenia than the biologic paternal half-siblings of control adoptees. This finding bolstered the hypothesis that schizophrenia is caused, at least in part, by genes.

Of course, there are some environmental correlates of the biologic parents that cannot be handled by the paternal half-sibling design. For example, children born to fathers of the lowest social class may share toxic environmental factors such as poor pre- and perinatal care, inadequate nutrition and an adverse social environment; these may confound the genetic parent–child relationship. This problem highlights a crucial inferential maxim of psychiatric genetics: *any conclusion about the role of genes and environment must rely not on a single study or class of study but on the converging evidence provided by a variety of research paradigms.*

Evaluating Adoption Studies

Like twin studies, adoption studies must be viewed with some caution due to potential methodologic problems that cloud their unambiguous interpretation. Perhaps the greatest limitation of adoption studies is the fact that adoptees and their families are not representative of the general population. The chain of events that lead parents to give up a child for adoption is complex and may be associated with the parents' (and hence the child's) genetic risk for psychiatric illness. For example, some teenage mothers who give up their children for adoption became pregnant due to impulsive behavior associated with drug or alcohol use. In many cases, the father may also be a drug user with sociopathic tendencies. Although not all adopted-away children have such parents, if the likelihood of having such a parent is greater for adoptees than for nonadoptees, then one cannot be sure that results from adoption studies will generalize to the broader population of nonadoptees.

This problem is further compounded by the fact that adoption may place particular stresses on the adopted child and his or her adoptive family. These stresses may increase the adopted child's risk for psychiatric disorders. Although we cannot be certain which of these factors are operative, research studies have confirmed that adoptees are indeed at greater risk for psychiatric disorders compared with nonadopted children.

The increased risk for psychiatric disorders among adoptees limits generalizability and demands that any psychiatric study of adoptees use an adoptee control group. For example, in the parent as proband study, the adopted-away children of ill parents must be compared with the adopted-away children of well parents. If we used the biologic children of well parents, the study would be confounded by the fact that adoptees are expected to have higher rates of psychiatric disorders than nonadoptees.

> **Key Point:** For studies seeking to determine the role
> of genes in causing disorders, it is not valid to com-
> pare adoptees whose parents had the disorder with
> nonadoptees whose parents did not have the disor-
> der. Such a comparison is invalid because adoption
> itself is a risk factor for mental illness.

Another problem is that it may be difficult to find a sample of
adoptees who were all separated from their parents at birth. If the child
has lived with a parent for even a short period of time prior to adoption, the biological relationship will have been "contaminated" by the
environment created by the child's biologic parents. Furthermore, the
environmental circumstances of parents may be associated with pre-
and perinatal events relevant to the etiology of the disorder under
study. For example, low social and economic status (SES) may be associated with poor pre- and perinatal care, resulting in environmental insults to the developing fetus and newborn. These must be considered
as environmental features that are difficult to disentangle from the genetic parent–child relationship. Some might even argue that the child's
contact with the mother immediately after birth creates a residue of environmental influence that effects subsequent psychopathology. Fortunately, such maternal influences can be assessed by using the paternal
half-sibling study.

SUMMARY: EPIDEMIOLOGIC FOUNDATIONS
OF PSYCHIATRIC GENETICS

In this chapter we described the three basic tools of psychiatric genetics: family, twin, and adoption studies. The family study is a systematic
extension of the clinical observation that a disorder appears to run in
families. By using a case–control study design, the family study investigator can provide a solid empirical foundation for asserting that a disorder is transmitted in families. Moreover, examining relatives with
varying degrees of genetic relationship can show if the pattern of transmission is consistent with the idea that genes underlie the familial
transmission.

The main strength of the family study is ease of use. In most clinics, assessing patients and their family members is straightforward. Interviewing all relatives in person can be time-consuming, but careful
interviews of appropriate family informants will yield meaningful data.

Yet, no matter how well designed, the family study method suffers one serious flaw: it cannot definitively disentangle genetic and environmental sources of familial transmission. For that task we must turn to twin and adoption studies.

The twin study capitalizes on nature's creation of monozygotic (MZ), or identical, twins and dizygotic (DZ), or fraternal, twins. Because MZ twins share all their genes with each other, any differences between them must be due to the environment. Like MZ twins, DZ twins share the same environment *in utero* and after birth. But, like ordinary siblings, DZ twins share only half their genes with each other. Thus, if genes cause a disorder, MZ twin pairs should be more likely to both have the disorder than DZ pairs. This allows researchers to parse the causal contributions of a disorder into three components: heritability (the fraction due to genes), shared environment (features of the environment common to twins), and unique environment (features of the environment not shared by twins).

> **Key Point:** Family studies are relatively easy to execute, but cannot disentangle the effects of genes and environment. Twin and adoption studies are difficult to execute, but can teach us more about the relative importance of genes and environment.

Like twin studies, adoption studies can disentangle genetic and environmental contributions to the familial aggregation of a disorder. They capitalize on the human institution of adoption which, for adoptees, creates two classes of relatives: biologic relatives, who influence them through genes alone, and adoptive relatives, who affect them through the environment. By examining the degree of transmission along biologic and adoptive lines, we can quantify the genetic and environmental contributions to etiology.

Although powerful methods for teasing apart the effects of genes and environment, twin and adoption studies have several drawbacks. Both are expensive and difficult to implement, for they require large samples of twins or adoptees with the disorder of interest. Moreover, adoption studies cannot be performed in some countries where access to adoption records is limited. Another problem is that twins and adoptees may not be representative of the general population or with clinical referrals, which makes it difficult to generalize findings from these studies. Finally, the results of adoption studies will be ambiguous if the adoptees were not separated from their biological relatives soon after their births.

Because each method has its limitations, we cannot rely on either a single study or class of studies to draw conclusions about the effects of genes and environment on mental illness. Instead, from an examination of many studies we seek a pattern of converging evidence that consistently confirms genetic and/or environmental hypotheses about the familial transmission of a disorder. When researchers have created this foundation of basic epidemiologic evidence they can then turn to variations of these basic designs to ask specific questions about genes, environment, and the causes of mental illness.

3

Variations on a Theme: Causal and Clinical Heterogeneity

All happy families resemble one another, but each unhappy family is unhappy in its own way.

—LEO TOLSTOY

*L*ike Kraepelin, Bleuler, Schneider, and other pioneering psychopathologists, contemporary clinicians are struck by the differing patterns of mental illness in the families of their patients. Mental illness riddles some families yet is rare in others. Sometimes family members share the same disorder; in other families, many disorders and mild, subclinical conditions are found. In short, a clinical perspective on families suggests that the familial nature of mental illness is heterogeneous as regards the types of illness transmitted and their severity in family members.

Figure 3.1 depicts the two dimensions of heterogeneity studied by psychiatric geneticists. *Clinical heterogeneity* occurs when more than one clinical condition can be brought about by the same cause; *causal heterogeneity* occurs when two or more causes can, on their own, lead to the same clinical syndrome;

Figure 3.1 shows that disease genes can lead to the three outcomes circumscribed by the large circle. Some individuals with the disease genes will have the "full disorder," by which we mean a clinical syn-

46

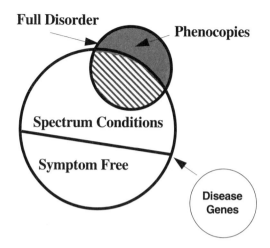

FIGURE 3.1. Causal and clinical heterogeneity. Adapted from Tsuang, M. T., Faraone, S. V. (1990). *The genetics of mood disorders,* p. 170. Baltimore: Johns Hopkins University Press. Copyright 1990 Johns Hopkins University Press. Adapted by permission.

drome that meets diagnostic criteria for a specific diagnosis; the small circle at the top of the figure represents people who have the full disorder. Others will not meet criteria for the full disorder yet will show the abnormalities we called "spectrum conditions;" the top half of the large circle represents these people. And finally, despite carrying the same disease genes as the affected cases, some individuals will remain symptom-free; the bottom half of the large circle indicates this group.

Thus, the figure shows how different phenomena can arise from the same genetic cause. This is called clinical heterogeneity. The disease called type 1 neurofibromatosis provides a dramatic example of clinical heterogeneity. Caused by mutations of a gene on chromosome 7, neurofibromatosis produces a wide range of symptoms. The "full disorder" is characterized by the extreme disfigurement of the body depicted in The Elephant Man, a successful Broadway play and Hollywood movie. But many patients are spared disfigurement and experience only mild changes to the skin.

The observation of clinical heterogeneity raises two additional questions: Why do two patients with the same genetic disease have such different outcomes? What mechanisms determine the difference? To answer these questions, scientists must piece together the pathway of events leading from mutant gene to clinical outcome. Somewhere along that path patients with differing clinical manifestations must differ either in their genetic makeup or in the environments to which they have been exposed. For example, the clinical heterogeneity of neuro-fibromatosis appears to be due, in part, to the nature of the specific mutation inherited and to the actions of other genes.

The small circle at the top of Figure 3.1 shows that not all cases of the full disorder are caused by the disease genes. Geneticists refer to cases falling outside the large circle as "phenocopies." These are cases of illness that mimic a genetic disorder but are not caused by genes. Alternatively, they may represent errors in diagnosis whereby a patient is diagnosed with a genetic condition but actually has some other disorder.

Phenocopies are a dramatic form of causal heterogeneity: some cases are caused by disease genes and others are not. In the simplest situation, the "other" cases are caused by some environmental event. Then it is sensible to posit genes as causing one variant of the disorder and the environment as causing the other. We must also consider the possibility that more than one set of disease genes can cause the same disease.

> **Key Point:** Psychiatric disorders have multiple causes, and the causes of disorders have multiple effects.
> Thus, when we use terms such as "schizophrenia," "depression," or even "Alzheimer disease," we are referring to a group of heterogeneous conditions.

Alzheimer disease provides a good example of causal heterogeneity. Three disease genes have been identified in families that have an early-onset form of the disorder transmitted in a dominant fashion: the presenilin-1 gene on chromosome 14, presenilin-2 gene on chromosome 1, and the amyloid precursor protein gene on chromosome 21. Notably, patients with each of these genetic defects show similar clinical features. We cannot tell which defect patients have based on their clinical presentations. Moreover, we cannot discriminate these genetic defects based on the condition of the patient's brain as determined by an autopsy: each of the genetic defects leads to the same type of brain abnormality. To make matters even more confusing, the clinical features and brain abnormalities seen in patients with these genes are also seen in other Alzheimer disease patients who do not have any of these genetic defects.

Remarkably, causal heterogeneity can occur within the same family. For example, in one family known to carry the presenilin-2 mutation that causes Alzheimer disease, two family members did not have the mutation but nonetheless had Alzheimer disease. It turned out that

TABLE 3.1. Questions and Answers for Family, Twin, and Adoption Studies

Questions of heterogeneity	Families holding the answers
Can we define genetic and nongenetic subtypes?	Families having one or more than one member with the disorder
Are there genetic variants of the disorder?	Families selected through a member having the disorder and families selected through a member who does not have the disorder
What are the neurobiologic correlates of genetic predisposition?	Families selected through a member having the disorder and families selected through a member who does not have the disorder
Do two or more disorders share familial causal factors?	Families selected through a member having one or the other disorder
Why do two disorders frequently co-occur?	Families selected through members having either or both disorders
How do we show developmental continuity between disorders of children and adults?	Families selected through a parent having the adult form or a child having the childhood form

these individuals had one of the other mutations known to cause Alzheimer disease.

Causal heterogeneity creates problems for researchers because there is often no way that clinical data can discriminate cases of illness caused by one set of genes from cases caused by other genes or by the environment. In Chapter 5 we will show how genetic linkage studies can discover different genes that lead to the same disorder. In this chapter we will limit our discussion of causal heterogeneity to the question: Can we discriminate disorders caused primarily by genes from phenocopies caused primarily by the environment?

This question is one of many raised by the heterogeneity of familial mental disorders. Clarifying causal and clinical heterogeneity is complicated by the fact that both may occur for any disorder. To deal with this complexity, researchers use several research designs, each of which answers a specific question about heterogeneity. You can think of each research design as describing the type of family that holds the answers to the questions of causal and clinical heterogeneity. Table 3.1 provides an overview of these questions along with the types of families we must query to find the answers.

To answer each question in column 1 of Table 3.1, the researcher must use the study design listed in column 2. A study design is a plan for comparing groups of families to answer questions posed by a researcher. The choice of design depends on the questions to be answered. You have already learned about three study designs in the preceding chapter: the case–control family study, the twin study, and the adoption study. Note that in Table 3.1, the word "families" refers to any type of family including nuclear families, extended families, twin-pairs, or adoptive families.

The following sections describe variations on family, twin, and adoption study designs used to answer the questions in Table 3.1, and provides illustrations from the scientific literature that show the value of these designs for clarifying the causal and clinical heterogeneity of mental illness.

CAN WE DEFINE GENETIC AND NONGENETIC SUBTYPES?

The question "Can we define genetic and nongenetic subtypes?" simplifies a complex question. As we discussed in Chapter 1, it makes no sense to describe some psychiatric disorders as genetic and others as environmental. Instead, genetic epidemiology seeks to describe both the genetic and the environmental contributions to disease. Nevertheless, we find it useful for some purposes to classify disorders as due primarily to genes or due primarily to the environment. For example, if you are seeking genes for depression, you would do well to start your search among families having a depression variant that is strongly influenced by genes. In contrast, if you plan to study how resilience to stress buffers some people from depression, you would do better to start your search with a primarily stress-induced form of the disorder.

> **Key Point:** Defining disorders as "genetic" and "nongenetic" is an idealization. It makes more sense to view the genetic and environmental contributions to illness as varying among people. By chance, some patients will have primarily genetic disorders and others will have primarily environmental disorders, but most are likely to have a mix of both types of causes.

Teasing apart primarily genetic from other forms of illness would also be useful for clinicians. As an example, consider a standard genetic counseling situation. A woman is contemplating having children but is concerned about her child's risk for depression given her own treatment for depression. Suppose we learn from patient interview that she had experienced an extreme grief reaction, had suffered only one episode of depression, and reported no depression among her relatives or her husband's. We would logically conclude that her depression was primarily induced by environmental factors, leading us to predict a relatively low probability of depression in her children. In contrast, if she had a history of multiple episodes of depression having no environmental precipitant and if she had several relatives with similar histories, we would view her depression as primarily genetic and estimate a higher risk for her children. Of course, few cases are so clear-cut, which is why some researchers have attempted to find clinical features that differentiate genetic and nongenetic subforms of illness.

The design used for separating primarily genetic forms from other subforms is straightforward. We find patients who have a family history of the disorder and call them "primarily genetic." Other patients we would classify as "primarily nongenetic." Ideally, we would select such patients from identical twin pairs. If only one twin was ill, we would classify that patient as having the primarily genetic form. If both were ill, we would define them both as having the primarily genetic form. In the case of schizophrenia, due to the rarity of identical twins with schizophrenia, researchers usually compare patients having one or more ill relatives with those having no ill relatives. Such studies provide useful data, but we must remember that this subdivision is prone to error: some patients with no family history of schizophrenia will still carry genes for the disorder.

The schizophrenia literature provides many examples of attempts to separate genetic and nongenetic subforms. Studies of these subgroups report some consistent results. Among patients with a family history of schizophrenia, researchers find deficits in the ability to attend to the environment, especially in a sustained fashion. In contrast, other schizophrenic patients are less likely to have problems with attention but more likely to show brain wave and brain structure abnormalities.

The structural brain studies are particularly interesting. They show that schizophrenic patients without a family history of the disorder are more likely than other patients to have large cerebral ventricles. These ventricles are empty spaces in the brain that fill with fluid. When brain atrophy occurs brain cells die off and create spaces between the remaining cells. Then the pressure of the liquid in the ventricles compresses this brain tissue, increasing the size of the ventricles to replace space once occupied by the atrophied nerve cells. Thus, the brain imaging studies suggest that there is less overall brain matter in brains of schizophrenic patients who do not have a family history of the disorder.

These results tempt us to conclude that brain atrophy in schizo-phrenia is due to environmental causes. This idea finds further support in a twin study by Dr. Daniel Weinberger and colleagues. They studied MZ twin-pairs who were discordant for schizophrenia: despite having the same genes, one co-twin had schizophrenia, the other did not. Such twin-pairs provide a lucid view of genetic and environmental causes of schizophrenia because the manifestation of schizophrenia in one twin must be due to some cause that differs between the twins. Because they have identical genes, that cause must be an environmental event. Thus, Dr. Weinberger reasoned that comparing the brains of ill and well dis-cordant twins would uncover the adverse effects of the environment that triggered schizophrenia in the ill twin.

As predicted, these researchers found more brain abnormalities among the schizophrenic co-twins compared with their unaffected co-twins. These results, along with other twin studies, suggested that some feature of the environment caused the brain abnormalities observed in schizophrenic patients.

Could it be that there are two distinct types of schizophrenia, one, showing brain atrophy, caused by the environment, and the other, not showing brain atrophy, caused by genes? If this were so, then there should be a subgroup of patients having enlarged ventricles that were clearly larger than the ventricles of other patients. But Dr. Weinberger and colleagues showed that, in contrast to this prediction, there was no clear distinction between patients with large and small ventricles. In-stead, they found that, among schizophrenic patients, ventricle size ranged from normal to abnormally large but there was no distinct point separating patients with normal and abnormal ventricles.

How do we harmonize these disparate findings? On the one hand, studies of familial and nonfamilial schizophrenic patients and of MZ twins discordant for schizophrenia suggest that there are qualitative dif-ferences between primarily genetic and other cases of schizophrenia. In contrast, we cannot demarcate a discrete group of patients having abnormally large ventricles, the putative marker for the primarily nongenetic form of schizophrenia. The reconciliation of these findings lies in the multifactorial model of vulnerability introduced in Chap-ter 2. Its suitability for schizophrenia was proposed by Dr. Irving Gottesman three decades ago. Dr. Gottesman proposed that schizo-phrenia did not have a single cause but was caused by the combination of many genes and environmental factors, each having a small additive effect on the expression of schizophrenia. This view is sometimes called the "multifactorial theory of schizophrenia" because it proposes that multiple causes lead to illness.

In the multifactorial view of schizophrenia, some patients have a primarily genetic form of the disorder because, by chance, they inherited many schizophrenia genes. Because they have many schizophrenia genes, it is likely that they will pass many of these on to their relatives. Thus, their high dose of schizophrenia genes makes it more likely that they will have relatives who also have schizophrenia.

In contrast, in some patients schizophrenia will be caused by a small dose of schizophrenia genes combined with exposure to a large dose of environmental adversity. These patients have a primarily environmental form of the disorder. Because these patients have a low dose of the causative genes, they will pass on a low dose to their relatives. Thus, their relatives will be at lower risk for schizophrenia than the relatives of patients who have a high dose of schizophrenia genes.

Although the multifactorial theory posits that it is possible to separate patients into groups with greater and smaller genetic contributions to their disorder, the fact of the matter is that most patients will fall between the two extremes of "primarily genetic" and "primarily environmental." This predicts that any measure believed to assess the effects of genes or environment will not separate patients into two distinct groups. Instead, it will have a graded distribution in the population. As we described above, this is exactly what Dr. Weinberger found for brain atrophy.

The multifactorial theory accords with studies that find differences between apparently genetic and apparently nongenetic forms of schizophrenia but cannot find a clear line of demarcation between the two. It does so by allowing the mix of genes and environment to vary among patients. At one extreme, some will have many predisposing genes and fewer environmental insults. At the other extreme, environmental assaults will explain most of the etiology. But most patients will have an equal mix of the two causal factors. According to the multifactorial theory, when we select patients having a family history of illness, we are more likely to choose patients from the "genetic" extreme, but we will also select many patients between the two extremes. Conversely, when we select patients who do not have a family history of illness, we are more likely to choose patients from the "nongenetic" extreme, but we will also select many patients between the two extremes. Thus, we will find differences between the two groups but will not see two distinct groups.

It seems that Dr. Gottesman was probably right: many or most cases of schizophrenia are probably caused by a multifactorial process. Nevertheless, researchers still pursue the possibility that other forms of schizophrenia may exist. These researchers are guided by the hypothetical breakdown of schizophrenia according to genetic and nongenetic types given in Figure 3.2.

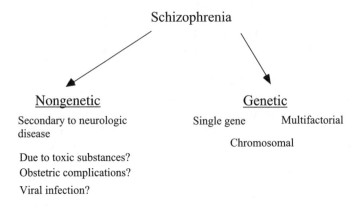

FIGURE 3.2. Genetic subtypes of schizophrenia.

The figure dichotomizes schizophrenia into genetic and non-genetic subtypes. Two of the nongenetic forms—those due to neurologic disease or toxic substances—would not, according to diagnostic convention, be given the diagnosis of schizophrenia. We include them only to remind the reader that schizophrenia-like syndromes can accompany neurological conditions (e.g., temporal lobe epilepsy), while others are caused by substances abuse syndromes (e.g., amphetamine psychosis). The figure also includes two speculative nongenetic forms. These derive from research suggesting that both obstetric complications and viral infection play a role in the etiology of some cases of schizophrenia. Although these two mechanisms appear to causally influence the onset of schizophrenic psychoses, it is unclear if they can do so in the absence of a genetic predisposition.

Dr. Sarnoff Mednick and colleagues provided a compelling example of how genes might combine with environment to cause schizophrenia. They proposed that brain atrophy among schizophrenic patients could be attributed to the effects of the genetic risk for schizophrenia in combination with obstetric complications. In their Danish study of children of schizophrenic parents, they showed that obstetric complications predicted brain atrophy, but only among children who, because they had a schizophrenic parent, were at genetic risk for schizophrenia. Thus, although it is tempting to search for purely genetic or purely environmental causes of schizophrenia, Dr. Mednick's work reminds us that a combination of genes and the environment might cause the disorder.

Figure 3.2 shows that cases of genetic schizophrenia probably fall into three categories. It is well known that rare forms of schizophrenia are due to overt aberrations of the chromosomes that are evident from laboratory tests (we describe such tests in Chapter 5). For example, some schizophrenic patients have extra sex chromosomes XXX and XXY. Others exhibit a variety of other gross anomalies of the chromosomes.

> **Clinical Tip:** The multifactorial model can be a useful tool for helping patients and their family members better understand the causes of mental illness. By emphasizing the role of environmental circumstances, you can show how psychosocial therapies can help people with mental disorders even though many of these disorders are believed to be biologically based conditions reflecting the dysregulation of brain systems.

A second group of genetic schizophrenia may be due to single gene defects. But, because the search for single major genes that cause schizophrenia has not yet been successful, these cases must be rare. The third and perhaps largest source of schizophrenia comes from Dr. Gottesman's multifactorial process. For these cases, several genes combine with one another and with environmental events to create a predisposition to schizophrenia. According to this model, no single factor is a necessary or sufficient cause for schizophrenia. Instead, if an individual's cumulative vulnerability exceeds a certain threshold, he or she will manifest the signs and symptoms of the disorder.

Later chapters will show how the multifactorial theory derives support from quantitative and molecular genetic studies. In this chapter we next show how the multifactorial theory explains the existence of mild, spectrum conditions that share a genetic etiology with psychiatric disorders.

ARE THERE GENETIC VARIANTS OF THE DISORDER?

As we discussed in Chapter 1, we use the term "spectrum conditions" to refer to mild psychopathology or other abnormalities of unknown clinical significance that occur among the otherwise well relatives of psychiatric patients. This term originated from clinical observations that found relatives of schizophrenic patients to suffer from a variety of schizophrenia-like conditions, for example, eccentric personalities, poor social relations, anxiety in social situations, and diminished emotional responses. Less frequently these relatives also showed mild forms of thought disorder, suspiciousness, magical thinking, illusions, and perceptual aberrations. These deviations were called "spectrum conditions" to convey the idea that the abnormalities form a dimension, or "spectrum," of pathology having schizophrenia at one extreme and subtle deviations at the other.

In research studies, some of the relatives exhibiting schizophrenia spectrum traits had gone past the usual age for the onset of schizophrenia. Thus, it seemed likely that their condition was not a *prodrome* to the disorder, that is, it would not eventually develop into schizophrenia. The crucial implication of this finding did not escape researchers: it appeared that schizophrenia was not a discrete condition. Instead, the discovery of spectrum disorders placed schizophrenia at the extreme end of a continuum of psychopathology.

This view of schizophrenia conforms to the concept of complex inheritance described in Chapter 1 (see Figure 1.1) and to the theory of multifactorial inheritance proposed by Dr. Gottesman. Both posit that each of us have been exposed to a set of genes and environmental insults that determine our susceptibility to developing a psychiatric disorder. This vulnerability cannot be directly measured so we can only describe it using hypothetical data, as in Figure 3.3.

As Figure 3.3 indicates, vulnerability is viewed as a quantitative or continuous trait. Most people have moderate levels of vulnerability, fewer have very high or very low levels. When a person's vulnerability exceeds the threshold denoted T_1, they will develop the full disorder. When it lies between T_1 and T_2, they will develop a spectrum condition. If it is below T_2, they will be unaffected and will not exhibit psychopathology.

We call Figure 3.3 a "multifactorial vulnerability model" because it assumes that many genes and environmental effects combine to create

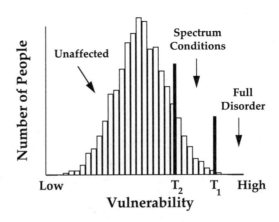

FIGURE 3.3. Multifactorial model of vulnerability.

any individual's susceptibility (this creates the bell-shaped or "normal" distribution of vulnerability). Unlike traditional medical nosologies, the multifactorial model eschews any qualitative distinction between those who have a disorder and those who do not have it. Instead, it posits that patients differ from nonpatients only in the number of pathogenic factors to which they have been exposed. In this view, we create a diagnostic rule by choosing a threshold (T_1) to separate patients from nonpatients. Such rules are useful conventions but, according to the multifactorial model, they should not be taken to mean that patients and nonpatients are categorically different, especially when we consider those close to the threshold of diagnosis.

> **Key Point:** The genes that cause psychiatric disorders also regulate a wide spectrum of traits. Some of these are mild clinical manifestations of the frank disorder; others can only be assessed using measures of brain functioning.

Some argue that the multifactorial model cannot explain discontinuities in the expression of psychopathology. For example, the psychosis of schizophrenia does seem categorically different from the illusions and magical thinking of a person with a schizophrenia spectrum disorder. So scientists have asked: Is there any way to make categorical and continuous phenomena compatible with one another? One answer to this question is the "mixed model" of vulnerability, described by the hypothetical distribution of vulnerability given in Figure 3.4. The mixed model allows for both multifactorial causes (which create much vari-

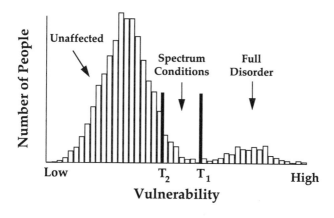

FIGURE 3.4. Mixed multifactorial model of vulnerability.

ability between people) and at least one large cause (which creates a distinct high vulnerable group). As Figure 3.4 indicates, like the multifactorial model the mixed model produces a continuum of vulnerability that is compatible with the existence of spectrum conditions.

Regardless of which model is correct, because both posit a continuous vulnerability to illness, many of their implications are similar. The clinical consequences of these models will not surprise many practicing clinicians. In clinical life we frequently face patients who are in substantial distress but do not meet the full criteria for any psychiatric disorder. These patients frequently meet all but one or two criteria and are thus considered subclinical cases. For some of these patients, psychiatric genetic data suggest that these mild syndromes are variants of clinically diagnosable conditions. In Chapter 6 we discuss the implications of such work for diagnosis and treatment.

For researchers, the vulnerability models suggest that etiologic or pathophysiologic studies of spectrum cases may shed light on the etiology and pathophysiology of the full disorder. Because the spectrum conditions are caused by fewer etiologic factors, the chain of events leading to their onset may be less complex, and therefore easier to understand. For example, the medications taken by some psychiatric patients have direct effects on the brain. Thus brain studies of patients sometimes cannot distinguish brain anomalies due to medication from those that underlie the disorder. In contrast, many people with spectrum conditions are not treated, so they can be studied without concerns that medication has caused brain abnormalities. Thus, the study of spectrum conditions provides researchers with a relatively clear window to study etiology and pathophysiology. If the vulnerability theory is correct, the view from this window should lead to insights about the causes of the full disorder.

How Do We Identify Genetic Spectrum Disorders?

Table 3.2 indicates the four criteria we use to identify spectrum disorders. The first criterion, *heritability*, requires that the trait is transmitted in families and that genes are known to play a role in its expression. If a trait is not heritable, then by definition it cannot qualify as a genetic spectrum disorder.

The second criterion, *familial link*, requires that "well" relatives of patients with the disorder express the trait to a greater degree than is found in the population at large. If the trait is only found among relatives who have the full disorder, then we would define it as a clinical feature of the disorder, not as a spectrum condition.

To meet the third criterion, *cosegregation*, the trait must be expressed by patients with the disorder either before, during, or between episodes

TABLE 3.2. Criteria for Classifying a Trait as a Spectrum Condition of a Disorder

Heritability	The trait shows familial transmission that is known to be due, at least in part, to genes.
Familial link	"Well" relatives of patients are at high risk for expressing the trait.
Cosegregation	The trait is seen among patients with the disorder either before, during, or between episodes of their illness.
Biologic and clinical plausibility	The clinical and biologic features of the trait are consistent with what is known about the disorder.

of their illness. For example, if an aberrant gene increases the risk for schizophrenia and also causes deficits on memory tests, then patients (who by definition carry the gene) must also show memory deficits.

The final criterion requires that the putative spectrum condition be *biologically or clinically plausible*. For example, if shoe size was thought to be a spectrum trait for schizophrenia and was shown to meet the first three criteria, we would remain skeptical because there is no plausible biologic or clinical reason why that should be so.

Because researchers have extensively studied spectrum conditions for schizophrenia, we will use this area of research as an example. This work has found two categories of spectrum disorders for schizophrenia: other psychotic disorders, and schizotypal personality disorder.

Psychotic Spectrum Disorders and Schizophrenia

The psychotic spectrum disorders are very similar to schizophrenia but they do not meet the diagnostic criteria necessary to make a schizophrenia diagnosis. Two prominent examples are "schizoaffective disorder" and "psychosis not otherwise specified" (NOS). As the name suggests, schizoaffective disorder is used for patients who exhibit features of both schizophrenia and affective disorders (also known as mood disorders). The affective symptoms of these patients include depression, irritability, and mania. In schizoaffective patients these symptoms are as prominent as the schizophrenic symptoms. In DSM-IV the diagnosis of schizoaffective disorder requires that an episode of mood disorder is present for a substantial portion of the psychotic episode. As the reader may surmise, patients are often classified in this category when the diagnostician finds an equal support for the schizophrenic and the mood disorder diagnoses.

Psychosis NOS is a residual diagnostic category. After we carefully apply diagnostic rules, we find that many of our psychotic patients do not meet the criteria for schizophrenia, schizoaffective disorder, or other psychotic diagnoses. The main identifying characteristic of psychosis NOS patients is that they have psychotic symptoms but do not fit into any more rigorously defined category. Using this category rather than forcing a choice between the more carefully defined categories is important. It reminds us that more information needs to be gathered to achieve diagnostic certainty. In many cases the psychosis NOS diagnosis serves as a temporary category for newly onset patients until the course of their symptoms reveals their diagnosis.

Both schizoaffective disorder and psychosis NOS are more common among the relatives of schizophrenic patients compared with the relatives of nonschizophrenic people. Thus, they satisfy our requirements for schizophrenia spectrum disorders. Curiously, schizoaffective disorder is also found among the relatives of patients with bipolar disorder. This has led some investigators to conclude that schizophrenia and bipolar disorder may share genes in common. In this view, the two disorders are at opposite ends of a "continuum of psychosis" and the schizoaffective patients lie in the middle. This controversial idea is now the subject of a good deal of research.

Another possibility is that some schizoaffective disorders are bipolar spectrum conditions and others are schizophrenia spectrum conditions. Notably, research has documented both depressed and bipolar subforms of schizoaffective disorder. Some genetic studies suggest that the depressed form is a spectrum condition of schizophrenia whereas the bipolar form is related to bipolar disorder. There is, however, some debate on this point due to the difficulties of making accurate diagnoses of schizoaffective disorder.

Personality Spectrum Disorders and Schizophrenia

The search for mild forms of schizophrenia started nearly a century ago when psychiatrists observed many relatives of schizophrenic patients to have "eccentric personalities." These relatives did not socialize easily with others, were anxious in social situations, and showed a limited range of emotion. The reader familiar with the diagnosis of schizophrenia will recognize that these symptoms are mild forms of schizophrenia's "negative" symptoms, observable or reportable features that indicate a loss of the normal range of activity, emotion, or cognition.

Clinicians also observed "positive" symptoms in the relatives of schizophrenic patients, including odd thought patterns, suspiciousness, magical thinking, illusions, and perceptual aberrations. These symptoms were similar to, yet milder than, the frank thought disorder, paranoia, delusions and hallucinations of schizophrenic patients. The mild schizophrenia-like symptoms seen in relatives of schizophrenic patients intrigued clinicians. Initially, some viewed these symptoms as signaling an impending schizophrenic episode. But because longitudinal studies eventually showed that most relatives with schizophrenia-like symptoms did not become schizophrenic, this idea was discredited. Instead, we now know that the syndrome of mild positive and negative symptoms seen in relatives usually does not change much throughout life. This syndrome emerges in childhood or adolescence and remains evident throughout the life cycle. To aid communication among clinicians and scientists, we now refer to this condition as "schizotypal personality disorder."

Schizotypal personality disorder is, in some ways, a milder form of schizophrenia. For example, schizophrenic patients will hear a voice when no sound is present; this is a *hallucination*. In contrast, schizotypal patients experience *illusions*, which are misperceptions of something, not perceptions of something that does not exist. For example, the sound of an air conditioner might be heard as a voice whispering. Schizophrenic patients often withdraw from society and isolate themselves to the point where they cannot effectively interact with others or their self-care is neglected. This avoidance of contact may be so extreme that they require hospitalization. The schizotypal person may also prefer to be a loner, but his or her withdrawal does not deteriorate to the point where the individual requires hospitalization.

Numerous family, adoption, and twin studies have documented the increased prevalence of schizotypal personality disorder among the biological relatives of schizophrenic patients. Thus, although there are some conflicting studies, there is general agreement that about 5–15 percent of the biological relatives of schizophrenic patients demonstrate nonpsychotic manifestations of schizophrenia. If even milder cases are included, nearly one-third of relatives may be affected.

Spectrum Conditions for Other Disorders

Although derived from schizophrenia research, the concept of spectrum conditions has proved useful for other disorders as well. Table 3.3 presents some examples. As the table shows, spectrum conditions are often clinically milder forms of the full disorders. These mild forms can be recognized disorders (e.g., schizotypal personality), but they can also be symptom clusters that would not qualify for a psychiatric diagnosis (e.g., negative schizophrenia-like symptoms such as restricted affect and social withdrawal).

TABLE 3.3. Examples of Spectrum Conditions

Disorder	Spectrum disorders
Schizophrenia	Schizotypal personality disorder Negative symptoms Neuropsychological impairment Eye tracking dysfunction Structural and functional brain abnormalities
Bipolar disorder	Hypomania Recurrent major depression
Panic disorder	Limited symptom panic attacks Behavioral inhibition
Autism	Anxiety disorders Social, communication, and cognitive deficits
Attention-deficit/ hyperactivity disorder	Depression Conduct disorder
Tourette syndrome	Other tic disorders Obsessive–compulsive disorder
Antisocial personality/ conduct disorder	Oppositional defiant disorder

In some cases, these relatively mild spectrum conditions might be final outcomes in the sense that some relatives with mild spectrum conditions will never express the full disorder; in other cases, the spectrum condition might represent a precursor or *forme fruste* of the more serious condition.

The distinction between outcome and precursor spectrum conditions is of much clinical importance in genetic counseling situations. For example, parents with a 26-year-old bipolar daughter will be concerned if they see hypomanic symptoms in their 13-year-old son because such symptoms are known to be precursor symptoms of bipolar disorder.

> **Clinical Tip:** Because spectrum conditions are associated with many disorders, it is likely that some relatives of your patients will have these traits. Thus, if the patient's family is involved in either the diagnosis or the treatment of the patient, family members' spectrum conditions may interfere with your goals. So be alert for these conditions and consider appropriate treatment as needed.

Although this section has focused on psychopathologic spectrum conditions, Table 3.3 indicates that the vulnerability to a disorder may be evident in direct or indirect measures of brain functioning. These measures are sometimes called "endophenotypes" because they cannot be observed or elicited through a psychiatric interview. We discuss endophenotypes in the next section, which shows how these conditions can clarify the relationship between brain dysfunction and the construct of vulnerability that we have used to explain the existence of spectrum conditions.

WHAT ARE THE NEUROBIOLOGIC CORRELATES OF GENETIC PREDISPOSITION?

In this section we show how the use of neurobiologic measures within a family study can find manifestations of a familial disorder in a manner that also clarifies its causes and associated brain abnormalities. We use the term "neurobiologic measure" to mean any assessment that directly or indirectly gauges the structure or functioning of the brain.

To understand the logic of a genetic neurobiology study, recall that most psychiatric disorders are probably due to the combined action of several genes and environmental factors. Thus, when families are selected through an ill member, for example, a schizophrenic patient, many of the nonschizophrenic members are likely to carry one or more schizophrenia-predisposing genes. If this is so, then these family members should display the brain defects caused by these genes. The goal of neurobiologic studies is straightforward: to detect such defects using measures designed to be sensitive to abnormalities of brain structure and function.

You may wonder why we would care to study brain abnormalities among the relatives who are *not* ill. Wouldn't it be more profitable to study the *sick* family members? Well, to fully understand the causes of a disorder we certainly do need to study patients. But, unfortunately, such studies can lead to ambiguous results because it is possible—some would say likely—that brain studies of frankly ill subjects are biased by effects secondary to the illness. For example, most patients with chronic schizophrenia have been exposed to years of neuroleptic drug therapy and many will have developed an alcohol or drug use disorder. We call these "secondary" effects because, rather than being direct manifestations of the illness, they emerge subsequent to its onset due to the necessities of treatment (in the case of neuroleptics) or the patient's response to her condition (in the case of substance abuse).

These secondary effects cloud the interpretation of neurobiologic tests. If, for example, a patient shows signs of cell loss in the brain, should we conclude that cell loss causes schizophrenia? Or was the cell loss caused by the use of licit or illicit drugs? We must also consider the possibility that psychotic episodes are themselves toxic and leave in their wake additional brain defects. Although we need to understand the causes of secondary brain anomalies along with their implications for treatment, we should not confuse them with the brain defects that caused the disorder.

Fortunately, these problems do not obscure studies of nonschizophrenic relatives because they have not received neuroleptic medication, most are not alcohol or drug abusers, and none have had neurotoxic episodes of psychosis. Thus, any abnormalities found among well relatives of schizophrenic patients can be attributed to one or more of the genes they share with their schizophrenic relative. If we assume that the effects schizophrenia genes exert on the brains of well relatives are similar to their effects on patients, then the study of relatives provides us with a view of the schizophrenic brain unclouded by the secondary effects of the disorder.

> **Key Point:** Because some relatives of patients carry the genes for illness but are not ill themselves, abnormal brain findings among relatives cannot be attributed to the illness or its treatment. Instead, such findings tell us about the effects that pathogenic genes have on the brain prior to the onset of illness.

As an illustration, we will describe observations of schizophrenia families completed by two of the authors (SVF and MTT) Dr. Larry Seidman and colleagues at Harvard Medical School. The first phase of this work relied on neuropsychologic tests, which require subjects to make written, verbal, or behavioral responses to a wide variety of problems. For example, a test of verbal memory asks the patient to recall ideas from a story. Tests of attention have the patient attend to a stream of letters and digits and respond when a specific combination occurs. From deficits in the performance of such tasks, neuropsychologists infer abnormalities in the brain systems believed to underlie the functions assessed by the tests.

We used neuropsychologic tests to examine brain functioning in 35 nonpsychotic adult relatives of schizophrenic patients and 72 normal controls. Figure 3.5 shows the neuropsychological scores of the relatives of schizophrenic patients. The scores for each neuropsychologic function were calibrated so that the average score for the controls was zero. For three functions, the relatives' scores dipped below zero to a

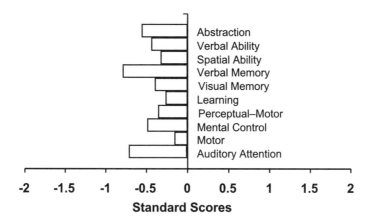

FIGURE 3.5. Neuropsychologic functioning among the nonpsychotic relatives of schizophrenic patients. A standard score of zero is normal performance. Negative numbers indicate below normal performance. Data from Faraone, S. V., Seidman, L. J., Kremen, W. S., Pepple, J. R., Lyons, M. J., & Tsuang, M. T. (1995). Neuropsychological functioning among the nonpsychotic relatives of schizophrenic patients: A diagnostic efficiency analysis. *Journal of Abnormal Psychology, 104,* 286–304.

degree that was statistically meaningful. Thus, we concluded that the relatives had deficits on those three functions: abstraction, verbal memory, and auditory attention. We were intrigued by these deficits because, although not as severe as those exhibited by schizophrenic patients, they were qualitatively similar. It was as if the relatives had a mild version of the severe neuropsychologic disorder seen in their schizophrenic relatives.

Because we did not study psychotic relatives, we concluded that neuropsychologic deficits among the relatives were not secondary effects of a psychiatric condition. Instead, they were probably due to one or more of the genes that had predisposed the family to schizophrenia. If that were so, we hypothesized that the deficits in neuropsychologic performance were probably due to abnormalities in the structure of the brain. If we could find these abnormalities, we would then have grounds for describing one piece of schizophrenia's pathophysiological puzzle: the piece provided by the genes that predisposed people to the disorder.

While we geared up for direct assessments of the brain among the relatives, we also decided to test another prediction of our theory: if abnormal genes caused the neuropsychologic deficits of the relatives, these deficits should be stable over time. Relatives who showed the deficits at the initial assessment should also show them if we tested them a second time.

Thus, we asked the relatives who had participated in our project to return for a second round of testing about four years after their original assessment. To simplify the analysis, we created a summary of the test scores that had discriminated relatives and controls at baseline. We found that this summary deficit score was reasonably stable over time. Figure 3.6 shows the results: subjects who did poorly at the original assessment (time 1 in the figure) tended to also do poorly four years later (time 2 in the figure).

Moreover, as we found at the original assessment, compared with controls, the relatives showed significantly worse performance on the summary score at follow-up. When we looked at individual tests we found that their problems in performance were clearly evident in tests of verbal memory and auditory attention. Additional tests implicated a cognitive function known as *working memory,* the mental function that allows us to keep information active in the brain for use in further mental processing.

In summary, our findings confirmed the idea that neuropsychologic dysfunction among relatives of schizophrenic patients is a stable trait, probably due to the gene or genes that had predisposed their family to schizophrenia. Given that these data were so encouraging, the next logical step was to directly examine the brains of the relatives us-

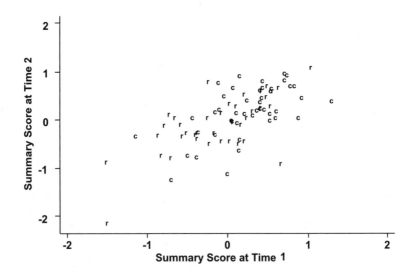

FIGURE 3.6. Summary scores at time 1 and time 2. r, relative of a schizophrenic patient; c, normal control.

ing the neuroimaging technology known as magnetic resonance imaging, or MRI for short.

MRI is one of several methods that allow us to visualize or "image" the structure and functioning of a person's brain. Although the method is exceedingly complex, its results are simple to understand. Put simply, the MRI takes a three-dimensional picture of the brain. From this computerized picture, we can estimate the size or volume of brain structures believed to be involved in the illness we are studying. The volume of a brain structure is a useful measure because deviations from normal volumes indicate aberrant brain development.

To assure a high-quality MRI scan, we arranged a research collaboration with colleagues at the Massachusetts General Hospital's Center for Morphometric Analysis. They imaged the brains of our subjects and computed the volumes of their brain structures. We show in Figure 3.7

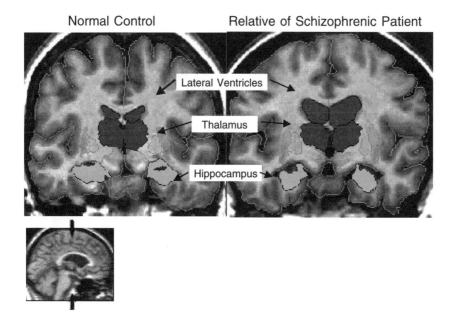

FIGURE 3.7. Structural brain abnormalities in a relative of a schizophrenic patient. These cases show brain slices imaged by MRI. They illustrate volume reductions in a relative of a schizophrenia patient compared to an age- and sex-matched control. The relative shows volume reductions in the thalamus and hippocampus and enlargement of lateral ventricles. Arrows on the small image indicate the position of the slice of the brain.

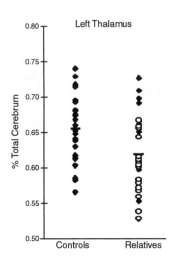
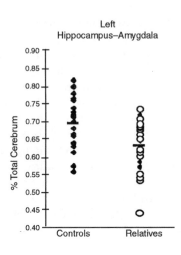

FIGURE 3.8. Adjusted volumes in selected brain regions. Regional volumes adjusted for total cerebral volume are contrasted in controls and relatives of patients. Compared with controls ($n = 26$), relatives of patients ($n = 28$) have reduced adjusted volumes in left hippocampus–amygdala ($t = -3.40$, $p < .0011$) and left thalamus ($t = -2.53$, $p < .014$). Horizontal lines indicate the mean adjusted volumes. Open symbols indicate siblings. Results were similar to structures on the right. Adapted from Seidman, L. J., Faraone, S. V., Goldstein, J. M., Goodman, J. M., Kremen, W. S., Matsuda, G., Hoge, E. A., Kennedy, D. N., Makris, N., Caviness, V. S., & Tsuang, M. T. (1997). Reduced subcortical brain volumes in nonpsychotic siblings of schizophrenic patients: A pilot MRI study. *American Journal of Medical Genetics, Neuropsychiatric Genetics, 74,* 507–514. Copyright 1997 L. J. Seidman. Adapted by permission.

an example of what they found. The figure shows—for one relative and one normal control—a single slice from the three-dimensional image of the brain. Three abnormalities are evident in the image of the relative's brain.

First, the structures labeled "lateral ventricles" are larger in the relative than in the control. These larger ventricles in the relative suggest that there is less overall brain matter in the relative's brain slice than in the control's slice. You can see the second abnormality by comparing the thalamus in the two images. The thalamus is somewhat smaller in the relative compared with the control. Because the thalamus is thought to play a crucial role in human emotions, attention, and memory, malfunction of this structure could conceivably predispose to the development of schizophrenia. A similar reduction is seen in the relative's hippocampus, a region that controls memory, one of the neuropsychologic functions known to be impaired in both schizophrenic patients and their relatives.

Of course, we cannot rely on the observation of a single relative and control to draw inferences about the brains of people related to schizophrenic patients. So we collected a larger sample of 28 nonpsychotic first-degree adult relatives and 26 normal controls. Compared with controls, relatives had significant volume reductions in the amygdala–hippocampus region, thalamus, and cerebellum. They also had significantly increased volumes in the pallidum.

Although the differences between relatives and controls were statistically significant, that is, not due to chance, they were small. This can be seen in Figure 3.8, which plots the individual left thalamus and left hippocampus–amygdala volumes separately for relatives and controls. Both graphs show that, although the relatives tended to have smaller volumes than the controls, there was still a good deal of overlap between the two groups. This makes sense from a genetic perspective. We do not expect all the relatives to have high doses of schizophrenia genes. By chance, some will have none and others will have many. Thus, we would expect that any putative measure of the effects of schizophrenia genes would show a range of normal to abnormal outcomes in the relatives.

Our MRI data suggest the hypothesis that abnormalities in limbic-diencephalic areas are core features of the genetic predisposition to schizophrenia. Because these relatives did not develop schizophrenia, the onset of the disorder must require other events that lead to further brain abnormalities and schizophrenic illness. This "event" could be another abnormal gene or exposure to a noxious environmental agent. These relatives did not have schizophrenia, so we cannot attribute their abnormalities to use of psychotropic medication or other secondary effects of the disorder.

> **Key Point:** The brain abnormalities found among relatives of schizophrenic patients show that their brains differ from normal, but they do not necessarily mean that the relative experiences any disability or distress. These abnormalities are "subclinical" in the sense that a radiologist reading most of these brain scans would not view them as clinically important. The more general point is that spectrum conditions may reflect one extreme of normal variation.

The brain regions implicated by our MRI studies play a crucial role in mediating emotional and cognitive behavior. Although more research is needed to clarify how brain abnormalities lead to specific defects, the regions we implicated could provide the structural underpinnings for the verbal memory, abstract reasoning, and attention dysfunctions we had found in relatives of schizophrenic patients. Supportive of this idea are data from other studies showing that damage to the thalamus frequently leads to problems of memory and attention. Damage to the hippocampus causes poor memory and may impair auditory attention. Moreover, dysfunction of anterior limbic structures, such as the amygdala, causes social–emotional deficits, which have also been observed in relatives of schizophrenics.

In summary, our neuropsychologic and brain imaging studies of schizophrenia families illustrate how family studies can be used to clarify the neurobiologic underpinnings of vulnerability. Although our illustration used the parents and siblings of schizophrenic patients, the method is easily generalized to other disorders and other family structures (e.g., twins and adoptive families).

DO TWO OR MORE DISORDERS SHARE FAMILIAL CAUSAL FACTORS?

The case–control study described in Chapter 2 yields definitive information about whether or not a disorder runs in families. It does not, however, tell us much about what is transmitted in families that have the disorder. In this section we describe a study design that answers the question: Is the observed familial transmission of a disorder mediated by genes or by environmental factors *specific* to the disorder? Or is it mediated by factors common to other psychiatric conditions?

We can answer these questions by studying three types of families: those selected through patients who have the first disorder of interest, families selected through patients having the other disorder, and families of normal controls. For example, because bipolar and major depressive disorders both involve mood dysregulation, and because both disorders run in families, many researchers have been intrigued by the possibility that the two conditions share causes that are familial.

This idea makes two clear predictions. Relatives of bipolar patients should have an elevated risk for depression and relatives of depressed patients should have an elevated risk for bipolar disorder. A thorough examination of this idea requires three types of study subjects: relatives of bipolar cases, relatives of depressed cases, and relatives of controls.

In fact, several studies have examined the prevalence of depression among relatives of bipolar disorder patients. Figure 3.9 shows the

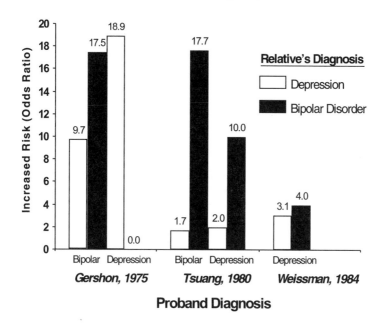

FIGURE 3.9. Studies examining the familial link between bipolar disorder and major depression. Data from Tsuang, M. T., & Faraone, S. V. (1990). *The genetics of mood disorders.* Baltimore: Johns Hopkins University Press.

increased risk for bipolar disorder and depression among relatives of bipolar and depressed probands. Each bar shows the increased risk in a specific relative group compared with relatives of normal controls. For example, the first bar shows that, in the study by Dr. Eliot Gershon, relatives of bipolar probands were 9.7 times more likely to suffer from a major depressive disorder compared with relatives of normal control probands.

As a group, the studies in Figure 3.9 show depression is two to ten times more likely to be found among relatives of bipolar patients than among relatives of control patients. These findings suggest that when depression occurs in bipolar families it shares familial determinants with bipolar disorder. Other studies have assessed the prevalence of bipolar disorder among relatives of depressed patients. These studies have been less conclusive. Some found about a fourfold increase in the risk of bipolar disorder among these relatives; other studies could not document any increase in risk.

The current thinking in psychiatric genetics is that when depression occurs in the family of a bipolar patient, it is likely due to some of the same genes that cause bipolar disorder. This is especially so if the depressed family member has had several episodes of depression. In contrast, depression in the absence of familial bipolar disorder may be very heterogeneous, with some cases sharing genes with bipolar disorder but others not.

> **Key Point:** Studies of two or more disorders can show if those disorders share familial causes, be they genes or environmental circumstances. The delineation of shared from nonshared risk factors is a crucial first step in planning treatment interventions to target specific disorders.

The search for specific and nonspecific familial factors can examine several disorders at one time. An example of this approach is the "Iowa 500" study of schizophrenia, bipolar disorder, depression, and normal controls conducted by one of the authors (MTT) and colleagues at the University of Iowa. The Iowa 500 study collected psychiatric interview data from 354 relatives of schizophrenic patients, 216 relatives of bipolar patients, 467 relatives of depressed patients, and 541 relatives of surgical control patients. This design allowed the investigators to answer several questions: Is schizophrenia familial? Is bipolar disorder familial? Is depression familial? and Are the familial factors causing these disorders independent from one another?

This latter question was of special importance. Nearly a century prior to the Iowa 500 study, Emil Kraepelin, the great German psychiatrist and, to some, the father of psychopathology research, posited schizophrenia and manic–depression (now known as bipolar disorder) to be separate entities. He based his assertion not on knowledge of etiology or pathophysiology (which was scant at the time) but on his observations of clinical features, course, and outcome.

Since both schizophrenia and mood disorders were known to each have a substantial genetic component to their etiology, the Iowa researchers devised a simple test of Kraepelin's idea: they sought to determine if the two types of disorders ran together in families. If mood disorders were simply a form of schizophrenia, then relatives of schizophrenic patients should show a high risk for mood disorders and relatives of mood-disordered patient should be at high risk for schizophrenia.

The results of the Iowa 500 study are given in Figure 3.10. As the figure shows, compared with relatives of controls, the relatives of schizophrenic patients had an increased risk for schizophrenia but not for mood disorders. In contrast, the relatives of mood-disordered patients had an increased risk for mood disorders, but not for schizophrenia.

The Iowa data, and similar reports from other researchers, suggest that Dr. Kraepelin was correct: schizophrenia and mood disorders appear to be separate entities that are unlikely to share a substantial amount of familial risk factors. When counseling families, information of this sort can be very useful. Many laypersons do not differentiate types of mental illness. Thus, when families inquire about the potential for a disorder to be transmitted in their family, data from such studies help clinicians communicate which disorders are likely to be transmitted and which are unlikely to occur. This latter information can be very comforting to people coming from families that suffer from relatively mild disorders like generalized anxiety. They will be relieved to know that they are not at risk for schizophrenia.

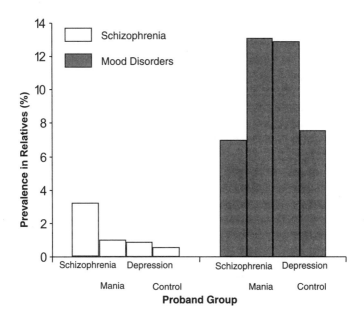

FIGURE 3.10. Prevalence of schizophrenia and mood disorders in relatives of schizophrenic and mood-disordered patients. Data from Tsuang, M. T., Winokur, G., & Crowe, R. R. (1980). Morbidity risks of schizophrenia and affective disorders among first-degree relatives of patients with schizophrenia, mania, depression, and surgical conditions. *British Journal of Psychiatry, 137,* 497–504.

WHY DO TWO DISORDERS CO-OCCUR?

Diagnostic manuals such as the American Psychiatric Association's *Diagnostic and Statistical Manual* (DSM) and the World Health Organization's *International Classification of Diseases* describe psychiatric disorders as separate illnesses. For example, early editions of the DSM endorsed a hierarchical approach to diagnosis. The DSM's diagnostic hierarchy told clinicians that if two disorders co-occurred, then the disorder higher in the hierarchy should be diagnosed. The disorder lower in the hierarchy was deemed a secondary condition of little clinical significance. For example, in DSM-III, panic disorder could not be diagnosed if episodes of panic were coincident with episodes of major depression.

As the DSM has evolved, many of its diagnostic hierarchies have been dropped so that clinicians can usually diagnose multiple disorders in the same patient. For example, in DSM-IV, panic disorder can be diagnosed even if episodes of panic are always coincident with major depression. The evolution of the DSM reflects both clinical experience and epidemiologic research: both suggest that psychiatric *comorbidity*—the co-occurrence of two or more disorders in the same patient—is a pervasive feature of mental illness.

> **Key Point:** A person having one psychiatric disorder has an increased risk for having other disorders. High rates of psychiatric comorbidity are found among community samples and clinical samples, among adults and children, and among men and women.

The comorbidity of psychiatric disorders will not surprise the working clinician: schizophrenic patients become depressed, depressed patients frequently have alcohol problems, alcoholics often abuse other substances, substance abusers often have ADHD, ADHD patients are likely to have learning disabilities, and so on. Of historical interest is the fact that these clinical observations were, for many years, attributed to "Berkson's bias," the fact that people with multiple disorders are more likely to seek help than those with only one disorder. The mentally ill seek help, or are brought to clinic by others, when they have reached an intolerable level of either psychological or emotional distress or psychosocial disability. Because people with two disorders are more likely to experience levels of distress or disability requiring referral, clinical samples present a skewed view of psychiatric comorbidity.

The use of the term "bias" is unfortunate because it has pejorative overtones and has led to confusion about the validity of research in clinical samples. Used in its narrow, statistical, and epidemiological sense, Berkson's bias means that when we estimate the fraction of depressed patients who drink too much in a clinic sample, our estimate will be higher than the "true" fraction, that is, the proportion we would estimate if we could examine every depressed person both inside and outside of our clinic. From this bias in the clinical estimate you should not infer that the clinical cases were incorrectly diagnosed. At a practical level this means that when you diagnose a patient with two disorders, that patient is probably not representative of the universe of possible patients, but that he or she probably has both disorders. For example, suppose that half of the depressed patients in your clinic are also alcohol abusers. Berkson's bias means that among all depressed people in the population, the frequency of alcohol abuse is likely to be lower. It does not mean that for any given depressed, alcoholic patient, one diagnosis is correct and the other incorrect.

To some clinicians, the idea of assigning a patient more than one diagnosis contravenes the principles of parsimony and differential diagnosis. After all, shouldn't the clinical alchemy of diagnosis transmute the comorbid patient's confusing conglomeration of symptoms into an unalloyed "true" disorder? This notion, that clinicians should distill a true disorder from a complex clinical picture derives from the hierarchical diagnosis paradigm that has guided research and clinical practice since the publication of DSM-III. This paradigm views psychiatric disorders as discrete entities that co-occur infrequently: some comorbidity is expected by chance, but for the most part, the presence of comorbidity signals diagnostic error.

The DSM's gradual move away from hierarchical diagnosis began when epidemiologists studied large population samples and found that comorbidity was not limited to the clinic waiting room. For example, the National Institute of Mental Health's Epidemiologic Catchment Area (ECA) study diagnosed thousands of people from several American cities. The ECA study found that, for psychiatric disorders, comorbidity was the rule not the exception. Figure 3.11 shows data collected by the ECA epidemiologists. The graph shows the increased odds of having other disorders for subjects with major depressive disorder. For example, the odds of having panic disorder were twenty times greater for depressed compared with nondepressed subjects. Depressives were also at greater risk for antisocial personality disorder, somatization disorder, substance use disorders, schizophrenia, simple phobia, and agoraphobia. Comorbidity was a pervasive feature of depression, not an error in diagnosis.

Because the ECA and subsequent epidemiologic studies of chil-

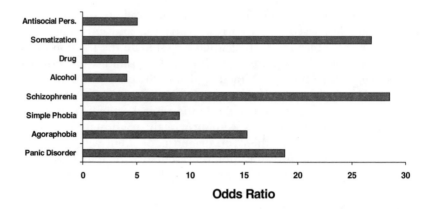

FIGURE 3.11. Increased odds of having other disorders for subjects with major depressive disorder. Data from Boyd, J. H., Burke, J. D., Gruenberg, E., Holzer, C. E., Rae, D. S., George, L. K., Karno, M., Stoltzman, R., McEvoy, L., & Nestadt, G. (1984). Exclusion criteria of DSM-III: A study of co-occurrence of hierarchy-free syndromes. *Archives of General Psychiatry, 41*, 983–989.

dren and adults found extensive comorbidity, clinical thinking—and the official diagnostic nomenclature—have moved away from hierarchical diagnosis and embraced the comorbidity paradigm. This paradigm views diagnostic overlap as the rule rather than the exception and encourages an empirical approach to diagnosis. By this we mean that the clinician assesses all disorders without assuming that some are primary and others secondary.

> **Clincal Tip:** Until research shows otherwise, if you are faced with a patient having two disorders, you should not routinely dismiss one as being secondary to the other. Instead, consider the implications each disorder has for treatment, course, and outcome.

There are two pillars to the comorbidity paradigm. First, *comorbidity is an empirical fact.* If we ignore it we place our patients in peril and impede scientific progress. The second point is equally important: *forced diagnostic choices can lead to diagnostic error.* Since diagnostic errors impede science and translate into treatment errors, psychiatric comorbidity is an urgent scientific and clinical issue.

Epidemiologic studies provide only one piece of the comorbidity puzzle: they show it is a valid phenomenon but cannot clarify why it occurs. As Table 3.4 indicates, many potential causes should be considered.

We should always consider the possibility that our nosology is sim-

TABLE 3.4. Possible Causes of Psychiatric Comorbidity

Cause	Description
Nosologic error	The diagnostic system is not correct.
Screening artifact	Comorbid disorders are more severe and more likely to be detected.
Diagnostic criterion overlap	Two disorders share diagnostic criteria.
Precursor syndromes	One disorder is an early manifestation of another.
Reporter bias	Patients with one disorder exaggerate the symptoms of another.
Secondary disorders	One disorder causes another.
Shared risk factors	Some risk factors for one disorder also increase susceptibility for another.

ply wrong. For example, if most dysthymic subjects also had major depression, and vice versa, it would not be sensible to consider their co-occurrence as comorbidity. It would make more sense to drop the distinction between the two.

An apparent comorbidity can be incorrect if it is based on a diagnostically weak screening test rather than a comprehensive diagnostic interview. For example, if we screen schoolchildren for psychiatric disorders by using teacher responses to rating scales, we will be likely to discover all of the severe cases but miss some of the milder cases. Because comorbid cases are usually severe, the teacher rating scale will overestimate the extent of comorbidity.

Diagnostic criterion overlap occurs because some disorders share diagnostic criteria with one another. For example, the diagnostic algorithms for both ADHD and depression include psychomotor disturbances and inability to concentrate. So, if a patient has ADHD, these two symptoms will make it easier for him or her to also meet criteria for depression.

Assessments of comorbidity must be attentive to the presence of precursor syndromes. For example, most children with conduct disorder will first meet criteria for oppositional defiant disorder. For these children, oppositionality may be viewed as the initial expression of the conduct disorder rather than as an entirely separate condition. A related idea is that comorbidity can occur when the early symptoms of two disorders are not distinguishable but, after a natural history unfolds, one can identify the true disorder.

Reporter bias occurs when patients with one disorder are biased to also report symptoms consistent with the diagnosis of another. For example, when diagnosing children, we often rely on reports from parents. It is possible that the experience of raising a child with one disorder, say ADHD, makes the parent more sensitive to the child's other behaviors, leading them to overreport symptoms of other disorders.

We must also consider the possibility that one disorder is a secondary manifestation of another. Although we have eschewed the idea that all comorbid conditions should be viewed in this manner, we must always consider this as a possibility. Some examples are clear: the patient with hallucinations caused by drugs or alcohol should not be diagnosed as schizophrenic. Others require considerable investigation: Is an alcoholic's depression secondary to the effects of alcohol? Is it a response of demoralization to a life of chronic psychosocial and occupational failure? Or does it indicate that the patient carries genes that predispose to depression?

Just as clinicians must tease apart the causes of comorbidity for individual patients, so must researchers disentangle cause from effect. Fortunately, several research strategies are available for this purpose. Symptom overlap studies assess comorbidity after adjusting diagnoses for overlapping symptoms. Follow-up studies determine if comorbid diagnoses predict course and prognosis. Multimethod assessment approaches use different methods of measurement to seek converging evidence for comorbidity. Multiple sampling strategies broaden the base of scientific inference by finding comorbidity in different types of samples.

Describing these methods goes far beyond the scope of this book. Instead, we focus on the family study and how it clarifies comorbidity by determining if and how comorbid diagnoses in a patient are transmitted among the relatives. The basic idea is that we can disambiguate complex, comorbid diagnoses in patients by examining the pattern of diagnoses in family members.

Figure 3.12 illustrates this idea for a single patient who meets diagnostic criteria for both major depressive disorder (MDD) and ADHD. Although the identified patient has two disorders, his brother and daughter are only depressed and his son only has ADHD. The finding of "pure" disorders in relatives cannot be attributed to another disorder and thereby supports the idea that this family suffers from two familial disorders which, by chance, both occur in the identified patient. By contrast, if there were no depression in the family but some members suffered from ADHD, we might conclude that the single case of depression was not familial and, perhaps, was secondary to the pa-

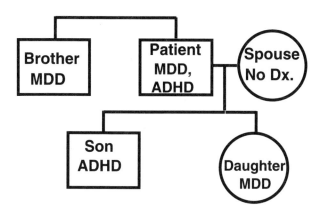

FIGURE 3.12. Schematic pedigree of comorbid disorders.

tient's ADHD. In a subsequent chapter we will discuss how clinicians can use family data to clarify individual patient diagnoses. In this chapter we address the issue of how the examination of many families can help us understand the causes of comorbid conditions.

When researchers examine comorbidity in families, they search for specific patterns indicating the presence of a mechanism that causes the two disorders to co-occur. The family study is a useful tool because it collect two types of people who have the disorder. We select families through probands who have the disorder. Because these probands are usually found in clinics, they are subject to artifacts that cause spurious comorbidity in clinically referred samples.

But we also examine the relatives of probands, many of whom will also have the disorder. Unlike the probands, these relatives are not selected for clinical referral. Thus, comorbidity among the relatives cannot be attributed to the artifacts that inhere in clinically referred case. Because families include both referred and nonreferred cases, we can use the pattern of comorbid disorders to make inferences about the genetic and environmental causes of psychiatric comorbidity.

We first consider the pattern predicted by the idea that referral artifacts cause comorbidity. If that is so, then we should find no cross-disorder familial transmission of disorders. For example, consider the well-known comorbidity between depression and anxiety disorders. Imagine that we selected probands with the following disorders: (1) anxiety only, (2) depression only, and (3) anxiety plus depression. If these disorders showed cross-familial transmission, then we should find anxiety and depression among the relatives of all three groups. In contrast, if the two disorders were independently transmitted in families, we should not find anxiety disorders among relatives of depressed-only probands and we should not find depression among relatives of anxiety-only probands.

As we will discuss later, a finding of independent transmission can have several interpretations, but if it is due to referral artifacts, we should find an additional pattern: we should observe psychiatric comorbidity among the probands, but not among the relatives.

Next consider another artifact that can cause comorbidity: misdiagnosis. Suppose that among patients with anxiety and depression, the diagnosis of depression is usually a diagnostic error. That might occur if the demoralization associated with a chronic anxiety disorder was confused with a true depressive disorder. If that were so, then a family study should find depression only among the relatives of depressed patients. The relatives of anxious patients and patients with both disorders should not be at risk for depression.

We have thus far given examples of how family study data detects spurious sources of comorbidity. But the power of the method reveals itself with the insights it provides into the mechanisms that cause comorbidity. Consider, for example, the well-established but poorly understood link between ADHD and learning disabilities (LD). When one of the authors (SVF) studied families of children who had both disorders, he and his colleagues found a high prevalence of LD among ADHD probands and their relatives. This could mean that some of the familial risk factors for ADHD also caused LD.

But, as Figure 3.13 shows, when they compared relatives of ADHD + LD probands with ADHD probands they found both groups of relatives were at risk for ADHD (the left panel of the figure) but that only the relatives of ADHD + LD probands were at risk for LD (the right panel of the figure). This pattern of ADHD and LD in families suggested that the familial risks for ADHD and LD were independent of one another because the apparent familial link between ADHD and LD was limited to families with LD probands. If the increased risk for LD had not been limited to ADHD + LD families, that would have supported the idea that the two disorders shared familial risk factors.

Further evidence for the familial independence of ADHD and LD was seen by examining the comorbidity of ADHD and LD among the relatives. As Figure 3.14 shows, having ADHD did not place the relatives at risk for having LD, that is, ADHD and LD did not show comorbidity among the relatives. The lack of comorbidity among relatives—despite the significant comorbidity among the probands—supported the idea that the two disorders were etiologically independent from one another and that their co-occurrence among relatives was due to an artifact.

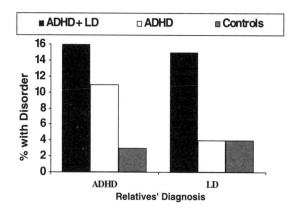

FIGURE 3.13. Prevalence of ADHD and LD among relatives of ADHD, ADHD + LD, and control probands. LD, learning disability; ADHD, attention-deficit/hyperactivity disorder. Data from Faraone, S. V., Biederman, J., Krifcher, B., Keenan, K., Moore, C., Sprich, S., Ugaglia, K., Jellinek, M. S., Spencer, T., Norman, D., Seidman, L., Kolodny, R., Benjamin, J., Kraus, I., Perrin, J., Chen, W., & Tsuang, M. T. (1993). Evidence for independent transmission in families for attention deficit hyperactivity disorder (ADHD) and learning disability: Results from a family-genetic study of ADHD. *American Journal of Psychiatry, 150,* 891–895.

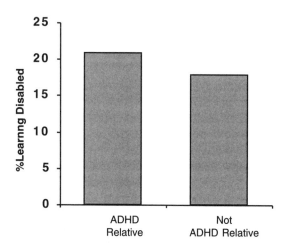

FIGURE 3.14. Independent transmission of ADHD and LD. Data from Faraone, S. V., Biederman, J., Krifcher, B., Keenan, K., Moore, C., Sprich, S., Ugaglia, K., Jellinek, M. S., Spencer, T., Norman, D., Seidman, L., Kolodny, R., Benjamin, J., Kraus, I., Perrin, J., Chen, W., & Tsuang, M. T. (1993). Evidence for independent transmission in families for Attention deficit hyperactivity disorder (ADHD) and learning disability: Results from a family-genetic study of ADHD. *American Journal of Psychiatry, 150,* 891–895.

At first this result might seem bizarre: after all, why would ADHD and LD be comorbid in the probands, but not in their relatives. One possibility was that children with both disorders might have been referred preferentially to our clinic. Yet that was unlikely because epidemiologic studies (which are not subject to this referral bias) also have found high levels of comorbidity. So, what was the explanation?

Well, it turned out that the comorbidity among the probands was due to nonrandom mating, which occurs when patients with one disorder show a tendency to marry and have children with patients who have another disorder. Figure 3.15 shows evidence of nonrandom mating between ADHD and LD. The graph shows the rates of LD in the spouses of parents who have a child with ADHD. We see the same result for both mothers and fathers. LD are more prevalent among the spouses of ADHD parents compared with the spouses of nonADHD parents. This significant nonrandom mating between ADHD and LD parents explains, in part, why some ADHD children have LD.

Figure 3.15 attributes the comorbidity between ADHD and LD to the intermarriage of ADHD and LD parents, not to risk factors common to the two disorders. As an example of this latter possibility, suppose that an aberrant D4 dopamine receptor was a component of the pathophysiology of ADHD and that the same were true for depression. Then children with ADHD would be more likely than average to have

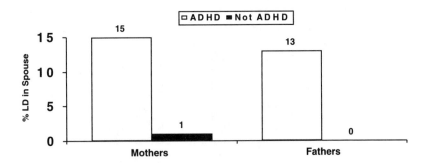

FIGURE 3.15. Nonrandom mating between ADHD and LD parents. Data from Faraone, S. V., Biederman, J., Krifcher, B., Keenan, K., Moore, C., Sprich, S., Ugaglia, K., Jellinek, M. S., Spencer, T., Norman, D., Seidman, L., Kolodny, R., Benjamin, J., Kraus, I., Perrin, J., Chen, W., & Tsuang, M. T. (1993). Evidence for independent transmission in families for Attention Deficit Hyperactivity Disorder (ADHD) and learning disability: Results from a family-genetic study of ADHD. *American Journal of Psychiatry, 150,* 891–895.

an aberrant D4 dopamine receptor gene, and would thus have a higher than expected prevalence of depression. Moreover, the relatives of ADHD children should also have an increased risk for depression, regardless of whether depression was manifest in the ADHD child. Conversely, we would expect depressed children and their families to have an increased risk for ADHD.

Thus, a minimum of two pieces of evidence are needed to assert that two disorders share common familial risk factors. First we must show that the two disorders occur together in families. As Figures 3.16 and 3.17 show, many studies have shown that this occurs for ADHD and depression. Children of depressed mothers are at high risk for ADHD (Figure 3.16) and relatives of ADHD probands have a higher than expected prevalence of depression (Figure 3.17). Although not all studies agree, when the studies are analyzed as a group using a method called meta-analysis, they show firm evidence for the idea that the two disorders co-occur in families.

Of course, as we saw for LD, artifacts can also cause disorders to co-occur in families. Thus, we must look for the second piece of evidence that favors the idea that the two disorders share familial risk factors: relatives of probands with ADHD should be at high risk for depression even if the ADHD proband does not have depression. As Figure 3.16 shows, we observed this pattern of familial co-occurrence in our data.

From the pattern of familial transmission shown in Figures 3.16 and 3.17, we have inferred that ADHD and depression share some familial causal factors, but we have not addressed another question: Why are some ADHD probands depressed and others not? One possibility is that patients with both disorders carry more of the familial risk factors needed to express each disorder. For example, perhaps depressed ADHD children carry more pathogenic genes than other ADHD children. If this were so, then the relatives of depressed ADHD children should be at higher risk for both ADHD and depression than other ADHD children. This makes intuitive sense. If you are related to someone who carries many pathogenic genes, your chances of having the disorder should be greater than if your relative carried few pathogenic genes. Thus, the "dose" of genes potentially transmitted by the proband determines the relative's risk for having the disorder.

But, as Figure 3.18 shows, our data do not support the idea that patients with ADHD and depression carry more pathogenic genes, or other familial risk factors, than do other ADHD patients. Thus, we must conclude that the difference between ADHD children with and

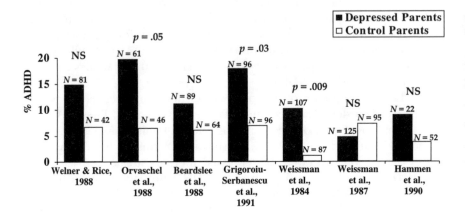

FIGURE 3.16. ADHD among children of depressed and control parents. Data from Faraone, S. V., & Biederman, J. (1997). Do attention deficit hyperactivity disorder and major depression share familial risk factors? *Journal of Nervous and Mental Disease, 185*(9), 533–541.

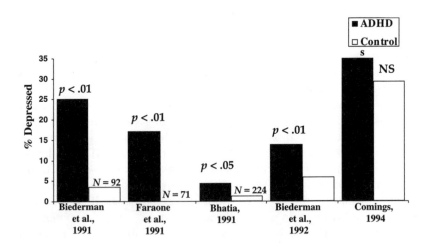

FIGURE 3.17. Depression among relatives of ADHD and control children. Data from Faraone, S. V., & Biederman, J. (1997). Do attention deficit hyperactivity disorder and major depression share familial risk factors? *Journal of Nervous and Mental Disease, 185*(9), 533–541.

without depression is due to some environmental risk factor that does not run in families. Examples of such etiologic agents include perinatal complications, head injury, and exposure to deviant peer groups. The pattern of disorders in families can implicate such causes but cannot determine exactly what that cause might be. To discover such causes we would need additional research projects that make measurements on putative environmental causes.

There is one more familial pattern of illness that can cause co-morbidity. This occurs when the comorbid condition is a genetically different disorder than one or both of the component disorders. We will use the example of ADHD and conduct disorder (CD). It is well known that about one-third of ADHD children show aggressive and antisocial behavior. It is equally well known that the siblings of ADHD children have an elevated prevalence of CD and that their parents show higher than expected levels of antisocial personality disorder.

As we discussed above, to better understand this apparent familial association, we must examine the risk to relatives separately for probands with and without the comorbid condition. Figure 3.19 shows the result: when we divided a group of ADHD probands into those with and without CD, the increased risk for CD was limited to those families that were selected through a proband who had both disorders. Being related to a proband who only had ADHD did not confer the familial risk for CD.

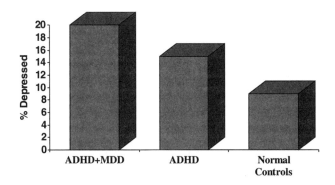

FIGURE 3.18. Depression among relatives of ADHD probands with and without major depressive disorder (MDD). Data from Biederman, J., Faraone, S. V., Keenan, K., & Tsuang, M. T. (1991). Evidence of familial association between attention deficit disorder and major affective disorders. *Archives of General Psychiatry, 48,* 633–642.

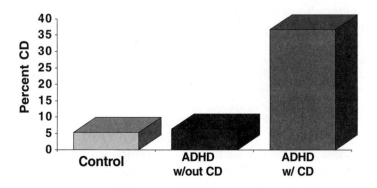

FIGURE 3.19. CD among relatives of ADHD and control children.

Because this pattern of familial transmission was consistent with the predictions of the referral artifact model, we also examined the second prediction of that model: If the comorbidity of ADHD and CD had been an artifact of referral, we should not observe comorbidity in the relatives.

If ADHD + CD probands carried two unrelated risk factors, one for ADHD and one for CD, ADHD and CD should be independently transmitted in the families of ADHD + CD probands. That is, relatives with ADHD should be at no greater risk for CD than those without ADHD. If, however, in the families of ADHD + CD probands, the degree of comorbidity in the relatives is greater than expected by chance, we use the term "cosegregate" to indicate that the disorders are transmitted together, not independently. That was the case in our data; there was a substantial degree of cosegregation. Among relatives of ADHD + CD probands, 49 percent of the relatives diagnosed as ADHD also had CD compared to 12 percent of the relatives who did not have ADHD. Such a finding could not be attributed to referral artifacts. Instead, it was consistent with the idea that the comorbid condition of ADHD plus CD was, from a familial perspective, distinct from other cases of ADHD. This suggests that ADHD with and without CD might have different etiologies and pathophysiologies and, perhaps, therapeutic responses.

> **Key Point:** There are several possible sources of psychiatric comorbidity. Current research suggests that much comorbidity reflects the actions of shared risk

> factors, but some cases of comorbidity can be attributed to artifacts of referral or patterns of marriage among people with mental illness. Much more research is needed in order to understand the causes of comorbidity and their implications for treatment.

Figure 3.20 summarizes the different patterns of familial transmission that family studies use to clarify the nature of psychiatric comorbidity. The figure uses ADHD and major depressive disorder (MDD) as examples, but the patterns presented apply to other conditions as well. We describe each model using a table with three rows, defined by the proband's diagnoses, and three columns, defined by the relative's diagnoses. The notation "+" predicts that relatives have an increased risk for the disorder labeling the column. The notation "++" indicates an even higher risk.

Panel A shows the expectations under a referral artifact model. For example, the first row shows that relatives of ADHD probands are expected to have an increased risk for ADHD but not for MDD. The second row predicts relatives of ADHD + MDD probands to be at increased risk for both disorders, and the third row shows that relatives of MDD probands are only at risk for depression. Put simply, each disorder is familial and there is no cross-disorder familial transmission.

You will see that the pattern of familial transmission predicted by the referral artifact model (Panel A) is also predicted by the nonrandom marriages model (Panel B) and the discrete subtype model (Panel C). But, as indicated at the bottom of each panel, we can determine which model is true because they differ in their predictions about comorbidity among relatives and random marriages of parents.

Panel D shows a misdiagnosis model that assumes that apparent cases of ADHD among MDD patients are misdiagnosed. If that were so, then we should only find MDD among the relatives of ADHD + MDD probands and MDD probands. We should find ADHD only among relatives of ADHD probands. We should not find much comorbidity among relatives (although some MDD relatives may be misdiagnosed as having ADHD), and there should be random marriages among ADHD and MDD parents.

Panel E presents the predictions of the familial dose model which assumes that the two disorders share a common pool of familial etiologic factors. Low doses cause either ADHD or MDD; at higher doses, both disorders occur. This model makes the straightforward prediction that the prevalence of ADHD and MDD should be highest among relatives of ADHD + MDD probands. Although these pre-

(A) Referral Artifact

Proband's Diagnosis	Relative's Diagnosis: ADHD	Relative's Diagnosis: MDD
ADHD	+	
ADHD + MDD	+	+
MDD		+

No comorbidity among relatives
Random marriages of parents

(B) Nonrandom Marriages

Proband's Diagnosis	Relative's Diagnosis: ADHD	Relative's Diagnosis: MDD
ADHD	+	
ADHD + MDD	+	+
MDD		+

No comorbidity among relatives
Nonrandom marriages of parents

(C) Discrete Subtype

Proband's Diagnosis	Relative's Diagnosis: ADHD	Relative's Diagnosis: MDD
ADHD	+	
ADHD + MDD	+	+
MDD		+

Comorbidity among relatives
Random marriages of parents

(D) Misdiagnosis

Proband's Diagnosis	Relative's Diagnosis: ADHD	Relative's Diagnosis: MDD
ADHD	+	
ADHD + MDD		+
MDD		+

No comorbidity among relatives
Random marriages of parents

(E) Familial Dose

Proband's Diagnosis	Relative's Diagnosis: ADHD	Relative's Diagnosis: MDD
ADHD	+	+
ADHD + MDD	++	++
MDD	+	+

Comorbidity among relatives
Random marriages of parents

(F) Nonfamilial

Proband's Diagnosis	Relative's Diagnosis: ADHD	Relative's Diagnosis: MDD
ADHD	+	+
ADHD + MDD	+	+
MDD	+	+

Comorbidity among relatives
Random marriages of parents

FIGURE 3.20. Patterns of familial transmission predicted by models of psychiatric comorbidity. ADHD, attention-deficit/hyperactivity disorder; MDD, major depressive disorder; +, high prevalence of disorder in relatives compared with relatives of control probands; ++, very high prevalence of disorder in relatives compared with relatives of control probands.

valences will be a bit lower when the proband has only one disorder, they will still be increased compared to what we would expect if the two disorders did not share familial etiologic factors.

The last model (Panel F), shows the expected pattern of familial transmission for the nonfamilial effects model. Like the familial dose model, this model assumes that ADHD and MDD share the same pool of etiologic factors. But, in contrast to the familial dose model, the model in Panel F assumes that the cause of the comorbid condition is some environmental agent. The model cannot determine the nature of the environmental effect, but from the predicted pattern of transmission we can infer its presence. The key feature of this pattern is that, unlike the familial dose model, comorbidity in the proband does not predict greater prevalences of either ADHD or MDD among relatives. Instead, relatives of ADHD, MDD, and ADHD + MDD probands each show, compared with the general population, an increased risk for both disorders.

HOW DO WE SHOW DEVELOPMENTAL CONTINUITY BETWEEN DISORDERS OF CHILDREN AND ADULTS?

Historically, child and adult psychopathology have been separate disciplines. Indeed, the professions have maintained this division by creating separate training programs for child and adult mental health clinicians. Specialty journals and specialized organizations cater to subspecialties defined by the developmental stage of the patient.

In many respects, this division is sensible. The biology and psychosocial milieu of childhood and adolescence are categorically different from their counterparts in adulthood. As they grow, children and adolescents experience continued brain development and hormonal changes while faced with psychosocial challenges unique to each stage of development. In contrast, by adulthood, the brain has fully developed, the hormonal assault of adolescence has subsided, and psychosocial challenges and stresses become less variable.

Moreover, the separation between child and adult psychopathology facilitates the creation of developmentally appropriate diagnoses and treatment approaches so that clinical work remains sensitive to the many changes that occur throughout the life cycle. But these somewhat separate traditions have led to ambiguities in diagnosis that can be addressed with genetic epidemiologic studies.

> **Key Point:** Studies of developmental continuity can
> determine if childhood disorders tend to remit, per-
> sist, or evolve into different manifestations during ad-
> olescence and adulthood.

Paramount among these ambiguities is the question of developmental continuity between child and adult disorders. Children and
adults differ in many ways but children become adults and childhood
conditions evolve into adult disorders. This leads to the question of developmental continuity: How are the clinical syndromes of childhood
transformed through development into the forms of psychopathology
observed in adulthood?

One method of answering this question is to perform a longitudinal study that follows children through childhood and adolescence into
adulthood. Such studies have provided much valuable data about developmental continuity. For example, they have taught us that ADHD children often grow up to be ADHD adults who are at risk for antisocial
personality and substance use disorders. Prior to these studies, ADHD
was a childhood disorder thought to remit by adulthood. The docu-
mentation of persistence into adulthood led to changes in the diagnostic nomenclature (which now recognizes ADHD as a condition of
adulthood) and corresponding changes in patterns of case identification and treatment in adulthood. Ongoing work by Russell Barkley and
others is now trying to determine if we should use different ADHD diagnostic criteria for children and adults. This makes sense, but how
does one go about deciding if a diagnostic algorithm for the adult version of a disorder is assessing the same disorder as the childhood version?

We will illustrate epidemiologic answers to this question with studies
of anxiety disorders because these present a complex spectrum of conditions throughout development. Studies of childhood anxiety disorders
consistently document different typical ages at onset for the various anxiety disorders. The anxious child will usually first experience a phobia of
animals, followed by situational-specific phobias, social phobia (in
midadolescence), and agoraphobia and panic disorder (in later adolescence or adulthood). This progression of disorders is accompanied by a
pattern of increasing psychiatric comorbidity with nonanxiety disorders.
Specific phobias have the lowest comorbidity, social phobia has intermediate levels, and agoraphobia and panic disorder have the highest.

Epidemiologic attempts to clarify the developmental sequence of
anxiety disorders have used two complementary strategies. The first examines the sequence of onset of disorders based on the retrospective

reports of anxious adults. The next prospectively observes the onset of anxiety disorders in children by examining them at several points through childhood, adolescence, and adulthood.

For example, retrospective accounts of the childhood histories of adults with panic disorder show that, when they were children, these patients often had separation anxiety disorder, social phobia, and overanxious disorder. A childhood history of these disorders is especially common among adults with severe early onset anxiety disorders complicated by psychiatric comorbidity. Thus, retrospective studies suggest that childhood anxiety disorders herald the eventual onset of relatively severe and complex anxiety conditions in adulthood.

Due to the expense of longitudinal studies, inferences about the developmental sequence of anxiety disorders have mostly relied on retrospective data, although one prospective study of subjects diagnosed with separation anxiety in childhood carried out by Dr. Rachel Klein and colleagues found these children to be at risk for the subsequent emergence of panic disorder and agoraphobia.

Compared with longitudinal studies, the family study provides a convenient but relatively inexpensive method of assessing the developmental continuity of disorders. The logic is straightforward: if phobias are childhood precursors of panic disorder, then children of panic-disordered parents should be at risk for phobic disorders. Likewise, the parents of phobic children should have an increased prevalence of panic disorder. Either finding would suggest that child phobias and adult panic are different expressions of the same familial condition.

To illustrate the genetic epidemiologic approach to developmental continuity, we will use a high-risk study of panic disorder that two of us (SVF and MTT) participated in at the Massachusetts General Hospital. The study (conducted by Drs. Jerrold Rosenbaum, Joseph Biederman, and Jerome Kagan) examined the prevalence of psychopathology among two groups of children. The first were selected through parents who had panic disorder. The second were control children whose parents did not have panic disorder.

As Figure 3.21 shows, compared with controls, the children of panic disorder patients showed significantly elevated rates of most anxiety disorders. Notably, 25 percent had two or more anxiety disorders and 7 percent had panic disorder. These results showed that the children of panic-disordered parents were indeed at high risk, not only for panic disorder and agoraphobia, but also for social phobia, overanxious disorder, and separation anxiety.

These results are notable from a developmental perspective because panic disorder and agoraphobia frequently co-occur and are commonly seen among adult psychiatric patients. In contrast, social

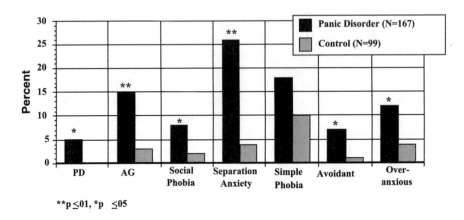

FIGURE 3.21. Anxiety disorders among children of panic disorder and control patients.

phobia, overanxious disorder, and separation anxiety are common disorders of childhood. Because the Massachusetts General Hospital family study showed that these disorders were associated across generations, it suggests that the childhood conditions may be an early manifestation of the adult disorders. Thus, it is reasonable to conclude that there is developmental continuity between the child and adult forms of these anxiety disorders.

> **Clinical Tip:** If you treat children and adolescents, be prepared for changes in a disorder's manifestation with development. In some cases, monitoring children with mental illness for the emergence of other disorders can speed treatment delivery and thus mitigate the potential effects of emergent disorders.

The data in Figure 3.21 raises crucial clinical questions: If the genetic predisposition to panic disorder can be detected at such an early age in the form of separation anxiety, social phobia, and other disorders of childhood, could we use these disorders to identify young children at risk for panic disorder? Could we then design preventive intervention programs for panic disorder? If so, how would we select patients for preventive treatments and what type of treatments would be appropriate? The nascent answers to these questions will be discussed in Chapter 7. But, before doing so, the next chapters will describe the mathematical and molecular genetics methods that will open new vistas for prevention research.

4

Mathematical Models of Inheritance

As far as the laws of mathematics refer to reality, they are not certain, and as far as they are certain, they do not refer to reality.

—ALBERT EINSTEIN

Mathematics may be compared to a mill of exquisite workmanship, which grinds your stuff to any degree of fineness; but, nevertheless, what you get out depends on what you put in; and as the grandest mill in the world will not extract wheat flour from peascods, so pages of formulae will not get a definite result out of loose data.

—THOMAS HENRY HUXLEY

*B*efore scientists understood the molecular basis of inheritance, they were able to describe in mathematical terms how genes would be expected to produce various patterns of inheritance in families. For several reasons it is crucial that we understand a disorder's pattern of inheritance, or "mode of transmission." This information can provide clues for subsequent research steps; for example, it would likely facilitate the discovery of genes through molecular genetic methods. Knowledge of inheritance patterns might also implicate environmental factors and provide clues to what these factors might be.

Describing the mode of transmission also facilitates genetic counseling, the process whereby clinicians inform individuals about the probability that they or their relatives will develop a genetic disorder. In the absence of a known mode of transmission (as is the case for most

93

psychiatric conditions), predicting genetic risks is relatively imprecise and must be based on empirical risk figures. Knowledge of the mode of inheritance would greatly improve the precision of such predictions.

MODES OF GENETIC TRANSMISSION

Single-Gene Inheritance

Before the discovery of genes, scientists and philosophers fiercely debated one another about how traits were passed from parents to offspring. Like many such debates, the question at hand was eventually resolved not by logical arguments but by the collection of data that consistently favored one theory over all others.

One might expect that the seminal discovery in genetics would have been made in a sophisticated laboratory at an esteemed university. One would be wrong: it was not. Instead, the story of modern genetics began over a century ago in the garden of a monastery where the monk Gregor Mendel (1822–1884), the father of modern genetics, tended pea plants. After observing the transmission of flower color and other physical features, Mendel devised clever experiments from which he harvested not only a fine crop of peas, but also the general principles of inheritance. These principles, which have stood the test of time, are now known as the laws of Mendelian inheritance.

> **Key Point:** The principals of single-gene inheritance are well worth studying. They are essential for understanding how scientists find genes, and they provide the biologic and mathematic foundation for complex modes of inheritance. Nevertheless, be alert to the fact that most psychiatric disorders are not caused by a single aberrant gene.

Today we know that there are two main types of single-gene transmission: dominant and recessive. It is easy to understand these two modes if you recall that we possess two copies of each gene, one inherited from our mothers, the other from our fathers. We say a disease is "dominantly inherited" if one copy of the disease gene can cause the condition. On the other hand, a recessive disease occurs only if we have two copies of the abnormal gene.

The patterns of inheritance have been inferred by studying the transmission of these conditions within families. This information can be expressed in the form of a pedigree, an example of which is given in Figure 4.1a. In a pedigree diagram, circles represent females and squares represent males. Filled-in symbols represent afflicted family members. A diagonal slash through the symbol means the family member is dead. Vertical lines connect parents and offspring, while horizontal lines connect siblings. Roman and arabic numerals indicate the position of individuals within the pedigree; roman numerals signify the generation and arabic numerals an individual within a single generation. For example, in Figure 4.1a, family member III-2 is a deceased female who had been affected; family member II-6 is a living male who is not affected but who has an affected sibling (II-7) and an affected father.

The pedigree signature of a dominant condition is its appearance in multiple consecutive generations. In this condition, both males and females are affected and both can pass on the disorder with equal probability. For example, in Figure 4.1a, affected individual I-3 had one son (deceased) and three living daughters. Two out of three of her daughters also are affected. Note that an unaffected individual (I-4) cannot pass on the disorder. The characteristic pattern of transmission is vertical, that is, the disorder is passed down from one generation to the next. Examples of this type of inheritance includes Huntington disease and some forms of Alzheimer disease.

To understand the dominant mode of inheritance we must consider what happens when paired chromosomes separate at the time of egg or sperm formation. As Figure 4.1b demonstrates, an affected father has one copy of the abnormal gene (A) and one copy of the normal gene (a). The father can pass either the normal or the abnormal gene to his offspring. Therefore, each child has a 50 percent chance of inheriting the disease gene (these are the "Aa" offspring in the figure). Each child also has a 50 percent chance of inheriting the normal gene and never developing the condition (these are the "aa" offspring in the figure).

Recessive disorders are conditions that are only expressed in people who have two copies of the disease gene. The characteristic pedigree pattern for recessive disorders is horizontal. By this we mean that coaffected parent–child pairs are rarely observed; the large majority of coaffected relatives are siblings. In Figure 4.2a, the half-filled circles or squares are unaffected individuals who carry one disease gene. For a child to have a chance of being affected, both parents must be disease gene carriers.

In Figure 4.2a, the parents (I-2 and I-3) are carriers and two of their children (II-4 and II-7) have inherited one disease gene from each parent and are therefore affected. However, because II-4 married an

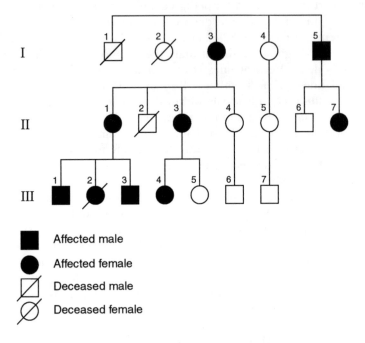

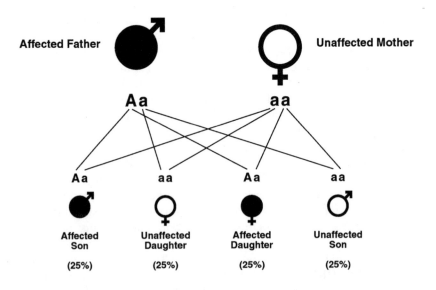

■ Affected male

● Affected female

⬦ Deceased male

⬦ Deceased female

FIGURE 4.1a. A pedigree of a family with autosomal dominant disease.

Affected Father　　　　　　　　**Unaffected Mother**

Aa　　　　　　　　　aa

Aa　　　　aa　　　　Aa　　　　aa

Affected　　Unaffected　　Affected　　Unaffected
Son　　　Daughter　　Daughter　　Son

(25%)　　　(25%)　　　(25%)　　　(25%)

FIGURE 4.1b. Transmission of an autosomal dominant trait.

unaffected individual (II-5) who has two copies of the normal gene, none of their children (III-1, III-2, III-3) are at risk for the illness. Common recessive conditions include cystic fibrosis and phenylketonuria.

People with recessive diseases usually have two carrier parents, as illustrated in Figure 4.2b. The two carrier parents (both with "Aa" genotypes) each have a 50 percent chance of transmitting the abnormal gene. By using probability theory, we can compute the chance they both will transmit the mutant gene to be 25 percent, which is the risk for two carrier parents to have an affected child. Using similar logic we can show that 50 percent of their children (the "Aa" offspring) will be unaffected but will carry the disease gene, and 25 percent (the "aa" offspring) will be unaffected children and will not carry the disease gene.

Typically, since carriers are relatively infrequent in the general population, these conditions do not occur unless parents are blood relatives. On the other hand, if the abnormal gene is frequent in a population (e.g., the cystic fibrosis gene, which is present in 1 out of 25 Caucasians), then children are much more likely to be affected even though the parents are not blood relatives.

In some cases, the pattern of transmission in families will be influenced by the sex of the family members. Notably, many psychiatric disorders show a differential prevalence in males and females. For example, males are more likely to be diagnosed with alcoholism, ADHD, and antisocial disorders, whereas females are at higher risk for depression and eating disorders. This sexual differential has led psychiatric geneticists to wonder if the genetic underpinnings of some disorders involve the two chromosomes, X and Y, that are responsible for sex determination. Although the degree of physical, psychologic, intellectual, and emotional differences between men and women can be the subject of vigorous debate, at the level of DNA the difference is undisputed: men have one X and one Y chromosome, women have two X chromosomes.

We call a disease "X-linked" if its genetic source involves genes encoded on the X chromosome. Such diseases have a characteristic sex distribution and pattern of inheritance. The hallmark of any X-linked disease is the absence of disease transmission from father to son. This happens because fathers only transmit a Y chromosome to their sons. Hemophilia-A and color blindness are examples of X-linked conditions.

As an example, consider the case of an X-linked recessive disease shown in Figure 4.3a. X-linked recessive disease pedigrees have a unique signature: all ill cases are male. The reason for this is simple: only males have the single X chromosome inherited from their mother. If it carries the aberrant gene, they cannot rely on the presence of a normal gene on another X chromosome to offset its effects. In con-

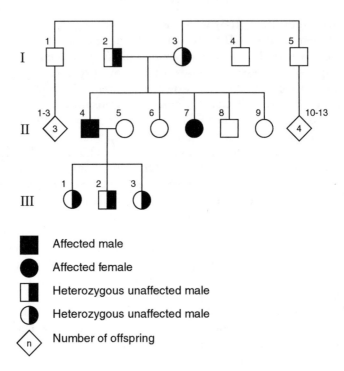

FIGURE 4.2a. A pedigree of a family with an autosomal recessive trait.

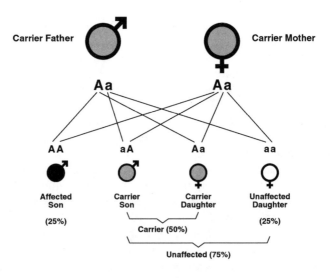

FIGURE 4.2b. Transmission of an autosomal recessive trait. A, abnormal gene; a, normal gene.

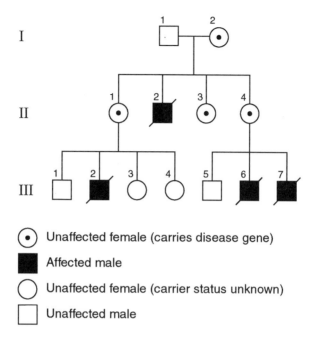

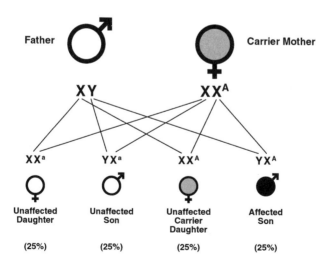

FIGURE 4.3a. A pedigree of a family with an X-linked recessive trait.

FIGURE 4.3b. Transmission of an X-linked recessive trait. A, abnormal gene; a, normal gene.

trast, females have the luxury of possessing two X chromosomes. If one carries a recessive disease gene, there is usually a good chance that the other will not. But females (such as II-1, II-3, and II-4 in Figure 4.3a) may carry the aberrant gene and can pass it on to their sons and daughters. These female carriers may pass either the normal or the abnormal X gene to either their male or their female offspring.

To understand X-linked inheritance, consider the mating patterns illustrated in Figure 4.3b, which shows that a woman having one normal and one abnormal gene has married an unaffected man. The carrier mother has a 50 percent chance of passing the abnormal gene to both her sons and daughters. However, only her sons can be clinically affected because her daughters have inherited a normal gene from their father.

Oligogenic Inheritance

Over 5000 human conditions are known to be inherited in a Mendelian fashion. More than half of these are dominant, about one-third are recessive, and less than 10 percent are X-linked. Unfortunately for psychiatry, simple patterns of Mendelian inheritance are not observed for mental illness. This makes it very difficult to determine the mode of inheritance for psychiatric conditions. We cannot simply "eyeball" a series of pedigrees and declare a disorder to be dominant, recessive, or X-linked.

> **Clinical Tip:** When patients inquire about the implications of their "genetic" disorder, they usually are under the false impression that their condition is inherited in the manner of well-known single-gene disorders like cystic fibrosis or Huntington disease. Thus, you will need to explain the basic principles of oligogenic and multifactorial inheritance to help them better understand the nature of their disorder.

Instead, as we have discussed in earlier chapters, the transmission of psychiatric disorders is likely to be oligogenic, or multifactorial. These modes of inheritance are usually referred to as "non-Mendelian." This nomenclature can lead to confusion because it incorrectly implies that the genes underlying complex diseases do not follow Mendel's laws. To avoid such confusion, just remember that when someone refers to a *disease* as non-Mendelian, he or she means that its pattern in pedigrees does not follow the pattern one would predict from a single gene. But the underlying genes follow Mendel's laws even if the associated disease does not.

Oligogenic inheritance occurs when the combined effects of a small number of genes cause a disease. Oligogenic genes can be either additive or interactive. We say that genes are *additive* if an individual's vulnerability to disease increases in direct proportion to the number of pathogenic genes he or she carries. Thus, for additive oligogenic diseases, someone having six pathogenic genes would have twice the risk for the disorder as someone having only three pathogenic genes. When genes are additive, the liability to disease can vary from low to high levels, depending upon the number of aberrant genes.

To complicate matters further, genes can combine in an interactive or an epistatic manner. *Epistasis* occurs when one disease gene (at a specific genetic location) determines whether or not a disease gene at another genetic location leads to disease. For example, we would describe a disease as epistatic if each of three disease genes were required for a disorder to develop. Someone inheriting any two of the three genes would not become ill. An illustration of this is Hirschsprung disease (a rare congenital condition that results in intestine immotility). One form of Hirschsprung requires the presence of two disease genes, one on chromosome 13 and one on chromosome 21. You will not develop Hirschsprung disease if you have one of these genes but not the other.

One difficulty in studying oligogenic models is that there are many ways in which genes might combine to cause a disorder. For example, there are 100 possible two-gene models that can describe a binary trait such as disease status. If the trait is trichotomous (either present, intermediate, or absent), there are over 2,000 possible models. A plausible argument can be made for excluding many of these possibilities because they either do not fit hypotheses about the disorder or they are biologically meaningless. Nevertheless, the number of models that remain to be tested is daunting.

Multifactorial Polygenic Inheritance

As we discussed in prior chapters, the multifactorial polygenic (MFP) model of inheritance proposes that a large, unspecified number of genes and environmental factors combine in an additive fashion to cause disease. The difference between oligogenic and polygenic models is one of degree. The former contain "several" genes (e.g., less than 10) whereas the latter include a "large number" of genes (e.g., 100). Polygenic models are used to describe continuous traits, for example, traits such as height and intelligence, that range from low to high and can take on many values.

We will illustrate the MFP model by starting with a single genetic location that can have one of two gene variants, A or B, coding for a trait (for this example, we will use height even though we know that it is not under the control of a single gene). Thus, any person's pair of genes must be AA, AB, or BB. We refer to a set of one or more pairs of genes as a "genotype." Rather than having some of these genotypes designated as "affected" and others as "unaffected," our hypothetical height genes produce different heights that increase with the number of B genes in a person's genotype. The AA genotype leads to a height of 120 cm, AB results in 150 cm, and BB leads to 180 cm. For this hypothetical example (where we assume that the A and B variants are equally common), the relative frequencies of heights among people with different genotypes is shown in Figure 4.4.

Now imagine that two genetic locations contribute to height. The genes at location 1 can be either A or B; at location 2 the choices are also A or B. Only B variants of each gene will increase height. This hypothetical model leads to the relative frequencies of heights illustrated in Figure 4.5. As the figure shows, very small people having the AAAA genotype are rare, as are very tall people having the BBBB genotype. In contrast, people with intermediate heights are more common.

In general, if there are n loci, then there are $2n + 1$ possible height values. In Figure 4.5, $n = 2$ and there are 5 possible phenotypes. As you can see, as the number of overall genetic loci increases, the closer the phenotypic distribution is to the smooth bell-shaped curve overlaid on Figure 4.5. This curve, known as the "normal distribution," fits well the population distribution of many traits believed to be controlled by polygenic inheritance.

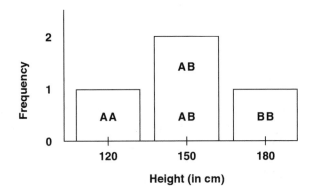

FIGURE 4.4. Hypothetical frequency distribution of a continuous variable (height): one genetic locus.

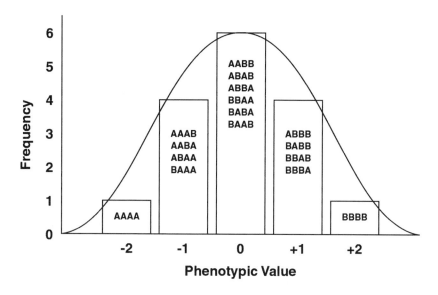

FIGURE 4.5. Frequency distribution of a continuous variable: two genetic loci. Data from McGuffin, P., Owen, M. J., O'Donovan, M. C., Thapar, A., & Gottesman, I. I. (1994). *Seminars in psychiatric genetics*. London: Royal College of Psychiatrists.

The concept of smoothly graded continuous traits makes intuitive sense for many physical and psychologic attributes such as height, weight, intelligence, and personality. Yet we usually view psychiatric disorders as dichotomous. You are either afflicted with schizophrenia or you are not. We are not accustomed to thinking that people have varying levels of schizophrenia.

A solution to this problem lies with the concept of spectrum conditions, which we have discussed in prior chapters. This concept views schizophrenia as a severe form of a condition that can also be expressed as schizoaffective disorder, schizotypal personality, or subclinical abnormalities in social functioning or neuropsychological performance. Even among schizophrenic patients, we can describe gradations of severity from the chronically ill hospitalized patient who is completely disabled through the relatively mild paranoid patient who may function well in a structured community setting. From a theoretical perspective, we can view these variant manifestations as being due to varying levels of schizophrenic "liability," even if we cannot assign a numerical liability score to each patient.

Thus, *liability* describes an unobservable characteristic in individuals which, under a multifactorial genetic model, is created by the additive action of disease susceptibility genes at many genetic locations. People with high levels of schizophrenic liability become schizophrenic, while those with lower levels develop other psychoses or other schizophrenia-related conditions in a dose-dependent fashion that varies with their "dose" of schizophrenia genes.

> **Key Point:** We use the term "liability" to refer to the underlying predisposition to develop a disorder. Liability is a hypothetical construct that cannot be directly measured. Instead, researchers who study multifactorial disorders seek to find the genes and environmental risk factors that combine to create the predisposition to illness.

But even if schizophrenic liability is a continuous trait, why are some people schizophrenic, others schizotypal, and still others unaffected? Within the MFP framework, the answer to this question has been the *liability threshold,* that point on the liability distribution that is large enough to cause disease. Thus, a multifactorial threshold model assumes that disease occurs when one's liability crosses a specific threshold. For example, perhaps there are 10 bipolar disorder genes and 8 are required for a person to become ill with that disorder.

Figure 4.6 illustrates the MFP threshold model. The top third of the figure shows two liability distributions: one for the general population (the thick line) and the other for first-degree relatives (i.e., parents, siblings, and children) of affected probands. The dotted line to the right of both distributions is the risk threshold. People with liability greater than the threshold become ill, those with a lower level of liability do not. The figure shows that first-degree relatives, who share half of the genes with an affected proband, have a distribution of genetic liability shifted to the right of the general population distribution. Their liability distribution is higher because, on average, they have more of the disease polygenes then does someone from the population. Second-degree relatives, who share a quarter of their genes with the affected individuals, will have a distribution that is closer to the mean of the general population (middle third of the figure). Third-degree relatives share only an eighth of their genes with a proband and have a liability much closer to that of the general population and therefore have only a slightly increased risk of developing the disorder (bottom third of the figure).

The threshold concept is also useful to describe spectrum condi-

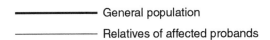

General population

Relatives of affected probands

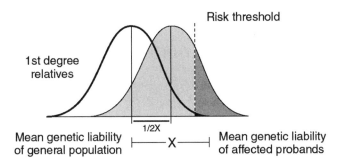

Risk threshold

1st degree
relatives

1/2X

Mean genetic liability
of general population

├———X———┤

Mean genetic liability
of affected probands

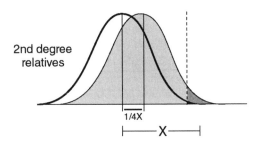

2nd degree
relatives

1/4X

├———X———┤

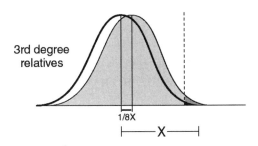

3rd degree
relatives

1/8X

├———X———┤

FIGURE 4.6. Genetic liability among first-, second-, and third-degree relatives. "X" denotes mean differences in genetic liability between affected individuals and individuals in the general population. Data from Gelehrter, T. D., & Collins, F. S. (1990). *Principles of medical genetics.* Baltimore: Williams & Wilkins.

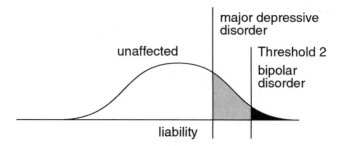

FIGURE 4.7. Two-threshold model for major depressive disorder and bipolar mood disorder.

tions because although these follow a gradient of severity, they are not—strictly speaking—continuously varying traits like intelligence. There is a clear and unmistakable demarcation between patients with schizotypal personality and those who are psychotic; there is no similar point of cleavage between people who have "superior intelligence" and those who do not.

To accommodate quasi-continuous traits such as spectrum conditions, more than one threshold may be placed along the liability continuum. For example, Figure 4.7 describes a multifactorial model used to investigate the genetic relationship between bipolar disorder and major depression. in Figure 4.7, individuals to the right of the right-hand threshold will develop bipolar disorder: those to the left of the left-hand threshold may have minor problems or be unaffected; those whose liability falls between the two thresholds would have an intermediate form of the disorder (such as major depression). Additional thresholds could be added to account for related conditions such as hypomania and minor depressive conditions.

SEGREGATION ANALYSIS: DETERMINING THE MODE OF TRANSMISSION

The term "segregation analysis" refers to mathematical methods used to determine the mode of transmission of a disease. Thus, given the correct type of family data, these methods will determine if a disease is transmitted in a dominant, recessive, X-linked, oligogenic, or multifactorial manner. They can also quantify the degree and nature of environmental effects, especially if twin-pairs or adoptive relatives are included.

A mathematical model of familial transmission translates assumptions about genetic and environmental causes into mathematical equations. These equations are then used to predict the distribution of a disorder that we observe in families or twin-pairs. If the pattern of disorder predicted by the model is close to what we observe, we say that the model fits the data. In contrast, if the predicted pattern of disorder differs from what is observed, we reject the model and seek another mechanism of transmission.

As the reader might suspect, the methods we discuss in this section require a good deal of mathematical and statistical expertise to understand and correctly implement. In the short space of this chapter we cannot present these mathematical details. Instead, we provide an overview of the different types of methods used to examine genetic and environmental transmission.

Overview of Mathematical Modeling

A genetic model comprises two major components. First, we must describe how the disorder is transmitted. For example, if we believe the disorder is due to a single dominant gene (a gene that will be expressed if one copy is present), our model must include the frequency of the gene in the population. It must also require that the transmission of the gene from parent to child follows Mendel's laws of genetic transmission. For example, if a mother carries one pathogenic gene, the probability that she transmits this gene to a child must be 50 percent.

> **Key Point:** The laws of genetic transmission can be described as mathematical rules. These rules are essentially probabilities that a gene variant will or will not be transmitted from parent to child. The simple mathematical rules of single-gene inheritance are used to create complex statistical models that can determine if the pattern of transmission of illness in a set of families corresponds to a specific set of genetic rules.

Models can specify environmental effects in several ways. Let's consider some simple examples. In a single-gene model we can specify the penetrance of each genotype. *Penetrance* indicates the probability that an individual carrying the disease gene will have the disease. If we believe that disease only occurs when an environmental event (e.g., head injury) occurs in someone carrying the pathogenic gene, then our model should allow some gene carriers to be unaffected (i.e., the disease gene is not completely penetrant).

For example, in one form of hereditary breast cancer, there is an age-associated penetrance risk in women who carry the susceptibility gene. In these families, the risk of developing breast cancer by ages 40, 60, and 70 is 20 percent, 54 percent, and 85 percent, respectively. Therefore, some unaffected women will have the susceptibility gene but will never develop breast cancer. The increases in risk with age could reflect aspects of the biology of aging, the cumulative impact of exposure to environmental toxins, or some combination of these or similar effects.

The second component of a genetic model is a procedure for determining whether the predictions made by the model adequately describe the pattern of illness observed in families. One modeling approach attempts to predict rates of illness in various classes of relatives. The family data are reduced to a table indicating the rate of illness in these classes (e.g., mothers, fathers, brothers, sisters, sons, daughters, and more distant relatives). The mathematical model is then estimated by choosing values for the model parameters (e.g., gene frequency and penetrance) that most closely approximate the observed rates. The observed and predicted rates can then be compared with a statistical test to determine if any deviation between observed and predicted rates is large enough to warrant rejecting the model.

Although useful, modeling rates of illness does not capitalize on all the information available in pedigree data. By lumping all families together within one data table, we cannot directly model the transmission of genes from one generation to the next. In contrast, pedigree analysis computes the likelihood of the pattern of illness in each family. For this approach the raw data are not summarized into a table. Instead, the analysis uses the status of each person and their relationship to others in the pedigree who are and are not affected. An algorithm then computes the likelihood that the assumed model is correct given the pedigree data and the value of model parameters. Those parameter values yielding the most likely model are used as final estimates. We then use a statistical test to see if this most likely or best model adequately predicts the pattern of illness in families.

For example, when we estimate parameters for a single-gene model we assume that a pair of genes at a single location or locus on a chromosome is responsible for the transmission of a disorder. If b represents the pathogenic version of the gene and B represents the normal variant at the same locus, then there are three possible genotypes: BB, Bb, and bb. Under Mendel's laws, the probability that a BB father transmits the b gene to his offspring must be zero. Likewise, the transmission probability that a parent of each genotype transmits B or b is fixed by the laws of Mendelian inheritance. This leads to a straightforward statistical test: compute the likelihood of a Mendelian model and compare this with a model that allows the transmission probabilities to deviate from their Mendelian values.

Unfortunately, segregation analyses in psychiatric disorders have not yielded consistent results. There have been many such studies of mood disorders and many of schizophrenia, but these have produced widely varying results and cannot be used to assert a certain mode of inheritance for either disorder.

Path Analysis

The method of path analysis was designed to partition-out effects of different genetic models and environmental influences. Path analysis aims to predict the relationship of variables under specified models. A path diagram is a useful tool to display causal paths among variables. The path model goes beyond measuring the degree of association or strength of relationships between two variables. Used correctly, path analysis can test hypotheses about causal relationships among variables quantified by the path coefficient.

In path analysis, causal relationships are diagrammed as we illustrate in Figure 4.8. In this model, four causes are used to account for the phenotypes of twins: unique environment (E), shared environment (C), additive genetic effect (A), and nonadditive (or dominance) genetic effect (D). The phenotype is either a continuous phenotype such as height or an assumed continuous liability as described above.

"Unique environment" refers to features of the environment not shared by siblings (e.g., they may have different friends). Any aspect of the environment not unique to twins is "shared" (e.g., they are raised under the same socioeconomic circumstances). Additive genetic effects occur when the effects of genes at each locus sum together to create genetic liability as we described in Figure 4.5.

The finding of nonadditive genetic effects could indicate that one or more disease gene loci show dominance. At these loci, there may be no difference between having one or two disease genes; either genotype equally increments the phenotype. Alternatively, two genes at different loci might interact with one another in an epistatic manner. These epistatic effects would also cause nonadditive genetic effects.

In path diagrams such as Figure 4.8, squares or rectangles represent observed (measured) variables and circles represent latent (unmeasured) variables. Single-headed arrows, or paths, are used to

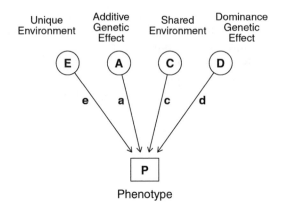

$$P = Ee + Aa + cC + dD$$

FIGURE 4.8. A path diagram demonstrating contributions of various genetic and environmental effects to a phenotype.

define causal relationships. Thus, in Figure 4.8, the observed trait P is determined by unobserved variables E, A, C, and D. The values next to the causal paths are path coefficients (e, a, c, and d). These estimate the strength of the effect of each corresponding causal variable (E, A, C, and D). The path coefficients can range from 0 (no effect) to 1 (a very strong effect accounting for all the variability in the phenotype).

A study by Dr. Robert McGue and his colleagues illustrates the use of path analysis. They examined two sets of family data: one described the familial transmission of schizophrenia, the other described the transmission of tuberculosis. Tuberculosis aggregates in families, like schizophrenia, but its etiology is known to be environmental. The estimates obtained from path analysis of schizophrenic families indicate a high and significant additive genetic effect ($a = 0.67$) along with a low and nonsignificant shared environment effect ($c = 0.19$). Estimates obtained from tuberculosis families were the reverse; the additive genetic effect was very low (0.06), while that of shared environment was high (0.62). Thus, using path analysis, investigators were able to correctly attribute the familial aggregation in tuberculosis to the environment.

> **Key Point:** Path analysis models can separate genetic from environmental effects. But to do so, they must include information from relatives outside the usual

nuclear family. Examples of additional relatives are twin-pairs, adopted children, spouses, and stepsiblings.

Path analysis is one of the most common methods for detecting environmental and genetic effects in families. A more complex model may also include assortative mating, cultural transmission, and maternal and paternal effects. For example, Dr. Kenneth Kendler and colleagues used path analysis to examined how parents transmit alcoholism to daughters. Figure 4.9 illustrates the best fitting model from an analysis of 1,030 female twin-pairs and their parents. This model included additive genetic (a) effects, individual specific environmental effects (e), and assortative mating (μ). Note that the genetic contributions was the largest ($a = 0.77$) compared to the other variables in the model: unique environmental effects ($e = 0.64$) and assortative mating ($\mu = 0.22$). This model estimated shared environmental effects to be zero, which led the authors to conclude that transmission of alcoholism from parents to their daughters was largely due to genetic factors.

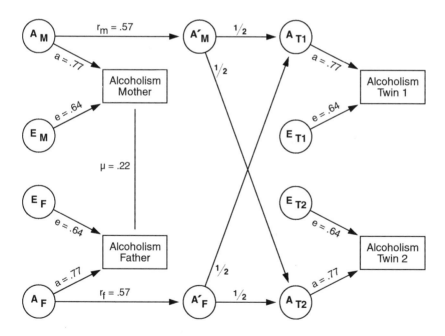

FIGURE 4.9. A twin-family model for twins and their parents. Path diagram demonstrating the best fitting model applied to alcoholism. From Kendler, K. S., Neale, M. C., Heath, A. C., Kessler, R. C., & Eaves, L. J. (1994). A twin-family study of alcoholism in women. *American Journal of Psychiatry, 151*(5), 707–715. Copyright 1994 by American Psychiatric Association. Reprinted by permission.

OBSTACLES TO ESTABLISHING THE MODE OF INHERITANCE

Despite the elegance and potential value of mathematical models of inheritance, these have not been able to unequivocally confirm a mode of inheritance for any psychiatric disorder. They have, however, provided many useful insights. For example, Dr. Irving Gottesman and colleagues used these methods to show that the transmission of schizophrenia could not be attributed to a single gene. Although subsequent work could not confirm an exact mode of inheritance, the falsification of the single-gene theory played a key role in orienting scientists to test additional hypotheses.

Likewise, mathematical modeling studies of twins have taught us much about the relative contributions of genes, unique environment, and shared environment. Notably, Drs. Robert Plomin and David Rowe and their colleagues have used mathematical models to highlight a counterintuitive finding that holds true for many psychological and behavioral traits: although the environment plays a key role in many of these traits, aspects of the environment that are common to siblings (e.g., social class, chaos in the family) are usually much less important than environmental features that are unique to siblings (e.g., exposure to peer groups, head trauma). These studies have led some to suggest that theories of developmental psychopathology may have overestimated the importance of the family environment in the pathogenesis of psychiatric disorders.

Mathematical twin studies have also confirmed an idea put forward by Dr. Sandra Scarr. She posited that our genetic makeup could lead us to choose our environments. For example, the genes that control anxiety and behavioral inhibition tend to make people avoid risks and not socialize much. In contrast, the genes that underlie novelty-seeking will lead to risk-taking and gregariousness. Unlike anxious people, novelty seekers will expose themselves to dangerous sports (which could cause head injuries), criminal activities, and a wide range of social situations. We intuitively categorize events such as head injuries as caused by the environment and we view social constructs such as "social support" as being features of the environment. Nevertheless, studies of twins show that these and other apparent environmental effects are actually mediated, to some extent by our genes.

Despite the valuable information provided by mathematical modeling studies, they have not been able to pin down the number of genes that cause any psychiatric disorder. There are two reasons for this failure. First, as the quote from Einstein at the beginning of this chapter elegantly states, "As far as the laws of mathematics refer to reality, they are not certain, and as far as they are certain, they do not refer to reality." The mathematical models of segregation analysis are certain inasmuch as they describe a mode of transmission in complete detail. They do not, however, refer to reality, which is much more complex.

In addition to the problems posed by the likelihood that many genes combine to cause mental illness, psychiatric geneticists must face additional obstacles. In general terms, genetically complex diseases do not exhibit a simple correspondence between the genotype (an individual's genetic composition) and their phenotype (an observable trait or disorder). As discussed in Chapter 3 (see Figure 3.1), this occurs when the same genotype causes different phenotypes (phenotypic heterogeneity) or when different genotypes can result in the same phenotype (genetic heterogeneity). Phenotypic and genetic heterogeneity have been inferred from many genetic epidemiologic studies of mental illness.

The analysis of complex diseases must also consider the possibility of non-Mendelian inheritance. One unusual example is mitochondrial inheritance. *Mitochondria*, the principle source of cellular energy production, are structures found in the cells of all organisms. They contain two types of DNA. Like all other cells in the body, their cells contain the DNA that constitutes our chromosomes. But unlike other cells, mitochondrial cells also contain additional DNA. This mitochondrial DNA occurs only in the mitochondria. The eggs of females contain mitochondria, but the sperm of males do not. Thus, only mothers transmit mitochondrial DNA to offspring. This leads to the peculiar pedigree signature of mitochondrial inheritance: affected individuals are always related through the maternal line, and no affected male transmits the disease.

Figure 4.10 illustrates mitochondrial inheritance by showing that only affected women (I-4 and II-2) transmit the disease; both their sons (II-3 and II-4) and daughter (II-2) can inherit abnormal mitochondria, but only the daughter can transmit them to her offspring. Abnormal mitochondrial DNA has been implicated in some rare neuromuscular diseases. Some scientists have suggested that mitochondrial mutations may be involved in bipolar disorder since excessive maternal inheritance has been reported in some families with that illness. However, because no specific mitochondrial mutations have been found in these families, this idea remains speculative.

The second problem for the analysis of complex traits is alluded to by Huxley in the epigraph which begins this chapter, an elegant statement of the less polished contemporary phrase "garbage in, garbage out." A mathematical model will not produce meaningful results if the psychiatric diagnoses it analyzes do not correspond to genetically crisp categories. The dilemma we face is that diagnoses were developed to

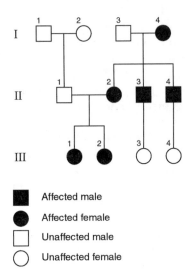

FIGURE 4.10. A pedigree of a family with mitochondrial inheritance.

serve many masters: clinicians, scientists, insurance companies, and more. There is no a priori reason why these categories should be ideal for genetic studies.

Because of the difficulties facing mathematical modeling studies, psychiatric geneticists have turned to molecular genetic methods. Although these methods also use mathematical procedures, they have one overriding advantage: their use of the family members' actual genes makes them powerful tools for discovering pathogenic genes. This powerful technology is the topic of our next chapter.

5

Molecular Genetics and Mental Illness

Only by strict specialization can the scientific worker become fully conscious, for once and perhaps never again in his lifetime, that he has achieved something that will endure.

—MAX WEBER

*I*n the prior chapter you learned how specialized tools from mathematical genetics can clarify how mental illness is transmitted in families. In this chapter we focus on the specialized technologies of molecular genetics, which have changed the way that scientists conceptualize illness and physicians treat its sequelae.

When scientists decide to search for genes that cause a mental illness, for example, bipolar disorder, all they know is that the disorder is inherited and that one or more of our approximately 80,000 genes must mediate its inheritance. But, it is not feasible to examine these genes one at a time, even if the search were to be limited to the approximately 30,000 genes expressed in the human brain. To make matters worse, genes constitute only about 2 percent of the 3 billion base-pairs of DNA that form our chromosomes.

Thus, a bipolar disease gene lurking among our chromosomes is the proverbial needle in a haystack. Remarkably, finding genetic needles in haystacks has now become almost routine for molecular geneticists; in fact, genetic diagnostic tests are now available for more than 450 genetic disorders. This chapter will describe how scientists find disease genes and explain what you need to know to understand published results from molecular genetic studies.

You may be wondering why you should bother to learn about molecular technology. Put simply, in the next decade, the ability to understand molecular genetic research will be needed to understand breakthroughs in the treatment and prevention of psychiatric disorders. Whether you read about these breakthroughs in scientific journals or the popular press, you will not know how they are relevant to your practice unless you have a basic understanding of their underlying methods.

If there is one fact you should take away from this chapter, it is this: the process of gene finding answers three questions about the nature of the gene and its implications for our patients. First we ask: *Where is the gene located?* To answer this question, we use linkage or association studies. These give us an approximate idea of where the aberrant gene lies, but they do not tell us which of the many genes in the implicated region is responsible for the disease. It was as if I told you that a million dollar treasure was buried in New York State. That information would help you to narrow your search, but it wouldn't make you rich any time soon without further information.

In genetics, that further information is provided by gene-finding technologies that answer the question: *Which gene causes disease?* In some cases the discovered gene may already have a known function; in others, its function may need to be divined by the scientists studying the disease. In recent years when the popular press has trumpeted news such as "Gene for Schizophrenia Found," it usually was referring to a linkage detection. In fact, as of this writing, with the exception of Alzheimer disease, none of the linkage detections for schizophrenia or other psychiatric disorders have led to the identification of a specific pathogenic gene.

> **Key Point:** Be careful not to confuse *gene detection*, the localization of a disease gene to a relatively small part of a chromosome, with *gene discovery*, the isolation of the disease gene and characterization of the mutations that cause disease. The path from detection to discovery can be long and difficult. Moreover, even when genes are discovered, it may take many years for scientists to understand how they cause disease.

After the gene has been found, another question must be answered: *How has the gene been disrupted to cause disease?* This is one of the ultimate goals of psychiatric genetics: if we can answer this question we will have a better understanding of the biological mechanisms that lead to disease and an improved framework for developing new treatments and preventive interventions.

The previous chapter described how mathematical models of inheritance provide valuable data about the mode of transmission and the relative prominence of genetic and environmental effects. These data are certainly useful, but they do not tell us which genes mediate transmission or how the environment combines with these genes to cause illness. To examine these issues, we must turn to molecular genetics.

In the late 1970s, following breakthroughs in molecular genetics, scientists recognized that it would be possible to identify a disease gene by locating its position on a specific chromosome even without knowledge of the gene's specific product or function. This process is called "positional cloning," or "reverse genetics." The term "reverse genetics" came into use because the process is, in a sense, logically backward. Instead of finding the biologic abnormality that causes disease and then using that information to find the disease gene, we first locate the gene and then examine its DNA in detail to determine its function and how it causes disease. This "backward" approach is especially useful for mental illness because we know so little about the biologic defects that underlie the signs and symptoms of illness in our patients.

The first success for reverse genetics came in 1983, when a segment of DNA on chromosome 4 was shown to predict Huntington disease within families. This was a remarkable feat: thanks to linkage analysis, a gene was detected without knowledge of its protein product or its biochemical action. Since then, more than 500 genes have been localized to specific chromosomal regions by using this strategy.

Another strength of reverse genetics is that the successful application of the method does not require us to know the disorder's mode of inheritance. Thus, if the methods of mathematical modeling fail to pinpoint a specific mode of transmission, reverse genetics can still find disease genes. Of course, before one starts any search for genes it is essential that prior evidence from family, twin, and adoption studies has confirmed that genes play a substantial role in causing the disease to be studied.

BIOLOGIC BACKGROUND

Before learning about how we find genes, it is essential that you understand the basic biology of inheritance. Every cell of our body contains genetic material carried by molecules called "chromosomes" (see Fig-

ure 5.1 for a schematic diagram). Humans have 23 pairs of chromosomes. One pair determines our sex: females have two X
chromosomes; males have one X and one Y chromosome. The other
22 chromosomes (called "autosomes") contain the genetic blueprint
needed to construct each unique person.

Each chromosome contains many million molecules of deoxyribonucleic acid, DNA for short. Each DNA molecule is built from four
"bases": adenine (A), guanine (G), cytosine (C), and thymine (T). As
Figure 5.1 illustrates, a DNA molecule consists of two long strings of
bases. The two strings are connected by the bases in a systematic manner: A is always paired with T and G is always paired with C. Thus, the
DNA molecule is a long string of base-pairs. Each of us is biologically
unique because, unless we have an identical twin, no other person has
the same sequence of base-pairs. Remember the adage "They broke the
mold when they made ____"? This is literally true for us all. Once we
are created, the probability that another nonidentical twin, human had,
has, or will have our exact sequence of DNA is infinitesimal.

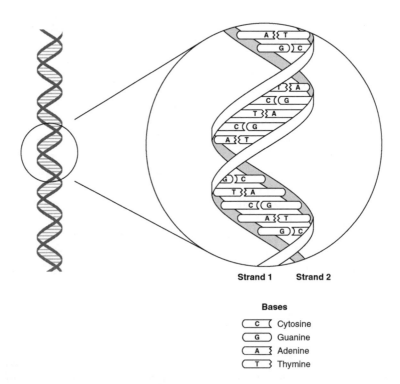

FIGURE 5.1. Schematic representation of a chromosome. Each chromosome is composed of one large DNA molecule.

So if chromosomes are made of DNA and DNA is made of base-pairs, where do genes enter the picture? Put simply, genes are segments of DNA that serve a biological function. As Figure 5.2 shows, because genes are segments of DNA they are built from a string of base-pairs. But for a base-pair sequence to pass muster as a gene, it must have some biological function—usually the creation of a protein that is needed for survival. Examples of proteins include hemoglobin in red blood cells that transport oxygen to all parts of the body and dopamine receptors that mediate neural transmission in the brain.

A mutation occurs when one or more of the base-pairs in a gene is missing or is replaced by another pair. In Figure 5.2, one of the T-A pairs in the normal gene has been replaced by a G-C pair in the abnormal gene. This base-pair substitution creates a mutated gene that produces a shorter protein, one that does not function correctly and leads to disease.

The work of molecular geneticists is complicated by two key features of DNA. First, only about 2 percent of our DNA actually contains genes. Some of the remaining DNA contains important base-pair sequences that regulate genes but most of it is "junk" DNA, which has no apparent biologic function but is suspected to serve as the raw material

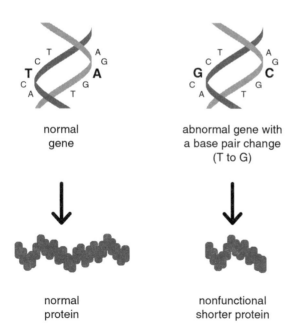

normal
gene

abnormal gene with
a base pair change
(T to G)

normal
protein

nonfunctional
shorter protein

FIGURE 5.2. Schematic representation of a gene and its protein product. A gene is a segment of DNA that makes a protein product.

for further evolution. So, when searching for the genetic needle in the haystack of 80,000 genes, scientists must also winnow through many sequences of junk DNA, which are much more common than the genes for which they are searching.

But molecular geneticists need to do more than simply find genes: they also need to determine how the normal sequence of base-pairs in a gene has been disrupted to produce disease. This brings us to the second complication posed by the structure of genes: on average, each gene is made up of 3,000 base-pairs. Obviously, finding which of these base-pairs is aberrant is no simple task.

Fortunately, the structure of chromosomes facilitates gene finding. They are composed of a protein scaffold formed by two strands of DNA intertwined to form a double helix (see Figure 5.1). Thus, chromosomes come in pairs and each member of a pair is itself composed of a pair of DNA strands.

Recall that the four bases that make up DNA (A, C, G, and T) are paired with one another, A with T and C with G. The two matched bases on opposite strands of DNA are called "complementary base-pairs." In other words, if the sequence on one strand is 5'-CGTAGGC-3', the other must be 3'-GCATCCG-5' (C pairs with G, G pairs with C, etc.). The notation 5'–3' (five prime to three prime) indicates the direction of the DNA molecule, with 5' designated as the leading end. The double-stranded structure can be written as

5'-CGTAGGC-3'

3'-GCATCCG-5'

As you can see, each DNA strand in a chromosome is the mirror image of its partner. Thus, each strand contains the full information content of the DNA molecule: if you know the base sequence of one strand, you can easily figure out the sequence of the other. At first glance, this redundant structure seems wasteful. Why did nature supply us with two strands when one contains all the necessary genetic information?

Although scientists invested many years of work in finding the answer to this question, it is surprisingly simple: when cells reproduce to create new cells, the double strand "unzips" itself and each complementary strand serves as a template for creating another DNA molecule. For example, if the two strands of DNA in the above sequence separate, the five-prime-to-three-prime strand serves as a template to create another three-prime-to-five-prime strand and vice versa. This works because the chemical nature of each base within a strand is such that it always prefers to be linked to its complementary base. Thus, a lone T on a single strand of DNA will attract any A bases that happen to be floating around the cell. Similarly, a lone C will attract a G, G's will attract C's, and A's will attract T's. After each base on each of the unzipped single strands captures its partner, there will be two sets of identical matching strands, that is, two identical chromosomes.

In cells, the ability of an unzipped DNA strand to find its correct mate in a mix of molecules is essential for reproduction. In the molecular genetics laboratory, this same ability is a useful tool for finding genes and understanding their function. Many molecular genetics techniques capitalize on this ability of a strand of DNA molecule to *hybridize*, that is, stick to its complementary strand.

As we previously discussed, a person inherits one member of each chromosome pair from his or her mother and one from his or her father. These inherited chromosomes, however, are not identical to either of the original parental chromosomes. During the formation of the egg or sperm, the original chromosomes in a pair may cross over with one another to exchange portions of their DNA. After multiple crossovers, the resulting two chromosomes each consist of a new and unique combination of genes.

Figure 5.3 illustrates the result of a single crossover. In this figure, the parental pair of chromosomes is represented by one dark and one light strand. One form of three different genes are represented on one chromosome with uppercase letters (A, B, and C); another form of each gene on the other chromosome is represented by lowercase letters (a, b, and c). The original pair of chromosomes on the left of the figure undergoes a single crossover in the middle of the figure. This

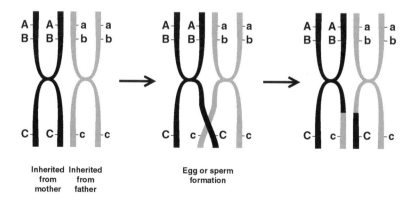

FIGURE 5.3. A schematic representation of a single crossover in a chromosome pair.

crossover exchanges one segment of DNA; the resulting chromosome pair is given on the right of the figure.

In Figure 5.3, the dark parental chromosome originally contained the genes A, B, and C and the light parental chromosome contained genes a, b, and c. After the crossover, two new strands are created: one contains genes A, B, and c, the other genes a, b, and C. These new strands will be incorporated into an egg or sperm. Thus, the chromosome transmitted to the child is not identical to the original parental chromosome. Moreover, Figure 5.3 presents a grossly simplified picture. In reality, many crossovers occur so that the final chromosome transmitted to the child is a hodgepodge of the parental pair.

Crossing over explains one of the many miracles of reproduction: *because we receive a jumble of genes from each parent, we resemble them in some ways but are in other ways different.* Crucial to this chapter is that crossing over also explains the molecular magic that finds genes in haystacks of DNA.

> **Key Point:** The crossing over of parental chromosomes within each parent creates new chromosomes that are transmitted to their children. This reshuffling of parental genes is the biologic basis of linkage analysis methods.

Consider first the chromosomes in the left panel of Figure 5.3. The genes A and B on the dark chromosome are close to one another and distant from C. Because there is not much room between A and B, crossovers will rarely separate them. In contrast, the large distance between B and C means that there is lots of room for crossovers to occur. Thus, A and B will tend to be transmitted together from parent to child, while B and C will be much less likely to be transmitted together. We say that two loci on the same strand are "linked" when they are so close to one another that crossing over rarely or never occurs between them (such as A and B). Closely linked genes usually remain together when they are passed on from parents to children.

On the other hand, distant loci (such as B and C) have a greater probability of ending up on different chromosomes. If two genes are on opposite ends of the same chromosome, there is a 50 percent chance that they will be transmitted together and a 50 percent chance that they will not. This is so because more than one crossover will occur between them. If the number is odd, they will end up on different chromosomes; if the number is even, they will be transmitted together. *As the physical distance between two genes decreases, the probability of them being transmitted together increases.* So if two genes are separated by half the length of the chromosome, the probability of being transmitted together is about 75 percent. If the distance between the two genes is one-fourth the chromosome's length, the probability for transmission is about 87 percent. If the distance is very small, such that the two genes are "linked" to one another, the probability of their being transmitted together is close to 100 percent.

To summarize: crossing over is the crucial biological event that allows us to find genes. It creates linkage among genes that are close to one another on the same chromosome. To capitalize on crossing over, scientists reasoned that family members having a genetic disease should be similar to one another on traits controlled by genes linked to the disease gene. For example, early studies of bipolar disorder found some families that showed no transmission of bipolar disorder from fathers to sons, which suggested that in these families a gene on the X chromosome might be causing the illness. Scientists also knew that color blindness was controlled by a gene on the X chromosome. The scientists reasoned that if a bipolar disorder gene was close to the color blindness gene, then, among families afflicted by both conditions, those family members with bipolar disorder should either *all* have color blindness or *all* have normal vision. That is, bipolar disorder and color blindness should be linked in these families. In fact, several investigators observed such linkage, leading them to conclude that a gene for bipolar disorder is resident on the X chromosome.

One aspect of the above example is worth repeating: if a bipolar disorder gene was located close to the color blindness gene, then, among families afflicted by both conditions, those members with bipolar disorder should either all have color blindness or all have normal vision. Note that there are two type of families. In some families, the parents who introduced the bipolar gene to the pedigree were color blind. They would contribute an X chromosome on which the bipolar disease gene was very close to a gene for color blindness. Because these genes would be transmitted together, most family members with the disease gene would have the color blindness gene and vice versa (we say "most" because even genes that are very close to one another will occasionally be separated by crossing over). In other families, the parents who introduced the bipolar gene to the pedigree were not color blind. They would contribute an X chromosome on which the bipolar disease gene was very close to a gene for normal color vision. Because these genes would be transmitted together (again, almost all the time), most family members with the disease gene would have the normal vision gene and vice versa. The key point here is that linkage between bipolar disorder and color blindness does not mean that bipolar patients are usually color blind. Linkage means that in some families they are usually color blind but in other families they are usually not color blind.

Although the above description is a bit simplified, it correctly conveys the main principle behind the process of genetic linkage analysis. If we can find a heritable trait with a known chromosomal location, then the co-transmission of that trait and a disorder can be used to determine if the genes controlling the trait and the disease are linked to one another. Having done so, the linkage analyst has collected extremely useful information: the chromosome containing the gene and the gene's approximate location on the chromosome. Later in this chapter we will discuss the statistical procedures used to determine if linkage exists and the laboratory procedures used to find and characterize the disease gene. But before doing so, we need to discuss another breakthrough of molecular genetics: the discovery of DNA markers.

DNA MARKERS FOR LINKAGE ANALYSIS

Although the method of linkage analysis had been available for many decades, its full power was stymied by the dearth of genetically mediated traits—like color blindness—that were needed to locate genes. Although some traits such as blood groups, enzymes, and human leukocyte antigens were useful to geneticists, they were not evenly distributed among the chromosomes. This meant that linkage analysts could determine if a disease gene was in one of several locations, but they could only examine a small fraction of the possible locations on the genome (i.e., our complete set of chromosomes).

Observable traits were also useless in families that did not express the trait. For example, one could not study the putative linkage between bipolar disorder and color blindness in families that were not afflicted by both disorders. Because most bipolar families do not have color-blind family members, it is not easy to recruit a sample of families large enough to detect linkage.

In the 1980s, molecular geneticists discovered a solution to this problem. Ironically, the solution lay in our "junk" DNA, those sequences of base-pairs that have no apparent biological function. After extracting DNA from blood samples, scientists learned how to describe small stretches of junk DNA. Because these small pieces of DNA had many variants at the same genetic locus, they were, like color blindness, an observable trait that marked a chromosomal location and therefore could be used for linkage analysis.

Moreover, these new DNA markers had two advantages. First, they were found throughout the genome. DNA markers are the milestones along our chromosomal highways. They are more or less regularly spaced at such small intervals that they allow linkage analysts to precisely localize disease genes anywhere along the genome. The second asset of DNA markers is their high degree of variability. In most families, several versions of the same DNA marker will be found in different family members.

An early example of a DNA marker was the restriction fragment length polymorphism, or RFLP. Scientists found that enzymes called "restriction endonucleases" could cut DNA into pieces at certain genetic sequences. The locations of the cuts were determined by the sequence of the nucleotides. For example, the restriction endonuclease known as AluI cuts DNA between the nucleotides guanine (G) and cytosine (C) wherever the nucleotide sequence AGCT occurs. The size of the resulting fragments is determined by the particular sequence of base-pairs at a genetic locus. For example, if one person has the sequence **AGCT**TGCTCTCTACC**AGCT**, AluI will cut out the fragment **CT**TGCTCTCTACC**AG**. If another person has the sequence **AGCT**TGCT**AGCT**ACC**AGCT**, AluI will cut out two fragments: **CT**TGCT**AG** and **CT**ACC**AG**. Thus, we can classify people according to the length of the fragment that results from cutting their DNA with AluI.

As discussed above, the ability of DNA markers to find genes improves with the number of marker variants that exist. This has led scientists to discover DNA markers with more variants per marker. One of these capitalizes on the fact that some base-pair sequences are repeated in tandem a variable number of times. These are called VNTR markers because they result from a variable number of tandem repeats. These hypervariable regions are usually 10 to 60 base-pairs long and consist of tandemly repeated sequences. The number of repeats varies among individuals from less than 10 to several dozen. Because differing numbers of repeats lead to different fragment sizes, there can be many variants at VNTR loci.

One type of tandem repeat DNA marker is the dinucleotide repeat in which two nucleotides (i.e., bases) such as CA or TG are repeated in tandem. At any specific locus, the dinucleotide may be repeated roughly 15 to 60 times. Tandem dinucleotide repeat markers are sometimes called "microsatellites." These markers have been especially useful since the number of base-pair repetitions vary a great deal among individuals, and can be easily tracked from parents to offspring. These markers appear quite frequently in the genome and provide a more efficient and rapid means for genotyping than RFLP markers. Moreover, the experimental procedures required to examine these markers are simpler than those required for RFLP type markers.

> **Key Point:** For genetic markers to be useful, they must be easy to measure and have many different variants at each genetic location. Contemporary DNA markers meet these criteria and are now widely used to find genes.

When scientists discover a DNA marker, they locate it on a genetic map, which shows its location relative to other DNA markers on the same chromosome. Each marker is assigned a numerical location, which is much like a mile marker on a highway. If someone tells you that she left a package for you at mile marker 385 on U.S. Interstate 80, you can easily find it. Similarly, if we learn that a gene is at DNA marker D10S1423, we have accomplished the task of gene location. The highway analogy is useful because it illustrates why we need many closely spaced DNA markers to find genes. If someone tells you that he left a package for you somewhere between mile marker 55 and marker 1,032 on Interstate 80, you may eventually find it but the task will be difficult. Obviously, the task of finding the package becomes easier as the distance between mile markers becomes smaller. Because this principle also holds for finding genes, molecular geneticists have created a very dense genetic map of DNA markers. These maps provide evenly spaced markers for genome wide scans.

STATISTICAL METHODS FOR LINKAGE ANALYSIS

Linkage analysis seeks to find chromosomal regions within families that tend to be shared among affected relatives but not shared among unaffected individuals. The regions are defined by the DNA markers that show statistical evidence of linkage in the analysis. Conceptually, linkage analysis takes place in three steps: (1) calculate a linkage statistic at each of many DNA markers (usually 300 or more) throughout the genome; (2) identify the markers which the linkage statistics show to be transmitted with the disease in families; and (3) test more markers in these regions of interest to more precisely localize the gene.

Consider a family with multiple blood relatives with bipolar mood disorder. First, markers are genotyped in all family members. By "genotyped" we mean that the laboratory determines which variants of the marker constitute the genotype of each family member. Figure 5.4 gives a hypothetical example of genotyping results in a family. Using the RFLP method, we cut the chromosomes into fragments that define a DNA marker at a known location. These fragments separate into distinct bands, as shown in the panel at the bottom portion of Figure 5.4. Each column in the panel contains DNA fragments for one family member.

To understand how the panel was created, consider the following analogy: It is as if each column was a cylinder containing a very viscous liquid. Because the fragments have different weights, if we pour them into the cylinder, the heavier ones will settle further toward the bottom than the lighter ones. We arbitrarily call these different fragment

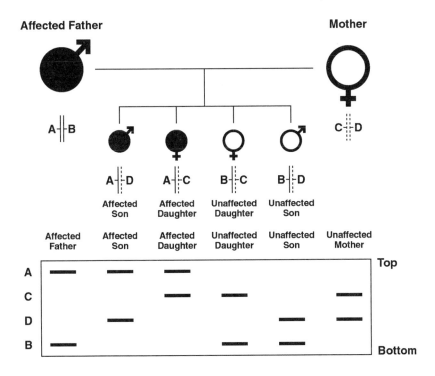

FIGURE 5.4. Genetic marker status from linkage analysis of an autosomal dominant condition. The bottom part of the figure depicts gel electrophoresis of DNA fragments after cutting with restriction enzyme; longer fragments (such as "B") settle at the bottom, while shorter fragments (such as "A") migrate to the top.

lengths, or "alleles," A, B, C, and D (different variants of the same gene are usually called "alleles").

In the upper portion of the figure, the affected father has allele A on one chromosome and allele B on the other, while the affected son has allele A and allele D. He must have inherited A from the father and D from the mother. The unaffected son has B on one chromosome and D on the other. He must have inherited allele B from his father. We see that affected children always receive the A allele from the father while the unaffected children receive the B allele. This suggests that the A allele is close enough to the putative bipolar gene so that the two are not separated during crossing over.

Given that the linkage between disease and marker seems obvious from Figure 5.4, you may be wondering why we need statistics to quantify our certainty that linkage exists. The answer is straightforward. In any real set of data, some families will be of the sort given in Figure 5.4, but others will give some evidence against linkage. For example, imagine that there was another family that had the same structure as the family in Figure 5.4 with one exception: the affected daughter inherited the B allele from her father. Thus, statistics are needed to summarize the evidence provided by a series of families in which some give evidence in favor of linkage and others do not.

We need statistical tests for another reason. When testing for linkage, we usually are uncertain about some aspects of the data. For example, the family in Figure 5.4 is easy to understand because the parents have four different alleles at the genetic locus being tested. But what if the mother did not provide a DNA sample and the sibship only included the two boys? We would not know for certain which alleles came from the mother and which from the father. We could, however, use a statistical model to tell us the most likely configuration.

The statistical theory underlying genetic linkage analysis is fairly complicated; so too are the computer algorithms that produce linkage results. Fortunately, these linkage analyses can usually be summarized in two crucial numbers: (1) a statistic whose magnitude increases with the evidence for linkage and (2) a number between zero and 1, which indicates the probability of computing the observed statistic in linkage was absent.

For example, some linkage analyses compute a Z-score for each DNA marker tested. On average, we would expect the Z-score to be zero for DNA markers not linked to the disease. But this is only the average we would expect from many markers. In reality, due to chance variations in our sample of families, some markers will have Z-scores greater than zero, which would suggest linkage.

> **Key Point:** Linkage analysis finds disease genes by showing that a genetic marker having a known genetic location tends to be transmitted along with the disease within families. We need to use statistical models to assure that the play of chance cannot explain any apparent excess sharing of marker variants among ill relatives.

Thus, we need a second number that will tell us the probability that any Z-score larger than zero would have occurred for DNA markers not linked to the disease. For example, if we computed a Z-score of 1.0 for a DNA marker, a statistical table would tell us that the probability of this score is .16, which means that there is a 16 percent chance that the magnitude of the Z-score is due to chance events, not linkage. By convention, nearly all scientists and statisticians would not conclude that the DNA marker is linked to the disease locus. The probability of that being the wrong conclusion is simply too high. In contrast, if the Z-score was high, say 6.0, then the probability of it being a chance event would be very low, about .000000001. Thus, this large Z-score along with its low probability value would give us a high level of certainty that the apparent linkage is real.

The Affected Pedigree Member Method of Linkage Analysis

This method is most easily described by referring to its most common form: the affected sib-pair study. The ideal sib-pair study recruits families in which two or more siblings have the disease of interest and are willing, along with their parents, to provide DNA samples. This method relies on our ability to infer "identity by descent" of DNA markers in siblings. We say that two alleles (one in each of two siblings) are identical by descent if both alleles were inherited from the same parent. For example, in Figure 5.4, the affected son and the affected daughter share one allele identical by descent (the A allele). In contrast, the affected son and the unaffected daughter share no alleles.

Because there are two alleles at each marker locus, we can describe a pair of siblings as having either one, two, or no alleles identical by descent at that locus. Now, suppose we collected 100 sib-pair families. Mendel's laws tell us that, on average, if a DNA marker is not linked to a disease, we should find 25 pairs sharing no alleles, 50 sharing one allele, and 25 sharing two alleles identical by descent. In contrast, if the DNA marker is linked to the disease, then pairs of ill siblings should be more likely to share alleles than is predicted by Mendel's laws. For example, in a series of 100 sib-pairs, a linked marker might show that 10 pairs share no alleles, 55 share one allele, and 35 share two alleles. In this series of families, sibs are more likely to share marker alleles than we would expect from Mendel's laws. But, we next ask, is the amount of sharing large enough to conclude that linkage exists? To answer that question we need the two key numbers already described: a statistic and its associated probability value.

The sib-pair method has been generalized in two ways. The affected pedigree member method is a general form of the sibling pair method. It allows all ill relative pairs to be included in the analysis. As is the case with siblings, linkage between a marker and a disorder increases the probability that any pair of ill relatives will share the same version of the genetic marker. A statistical algorithm then determines if the amount of marker sharing is greater than what one would expect by chance alone.

The affected pedigree member method can also be used when identity by descent cannot be established with certainty. For example, consider two siblings. The first carries the marker alleles A and B, the second marker alleles A and C. Now assume their father's genotype is AC but that the mother's genotype is unknown because she did not provide a DNA sample. We can infer from the first sib's genotype (AB) that, because the father carries A and C, the mother must have had the B allele, so the first sib must have inherited A from his father. But the second sib is ambiguous. She may have inherited the A allele from her father and C from her mother or vice versa. Thus, we can conclude that the two siblings' A alleles are identical by state (i.e., they are the same version of the DNA marker) but we cannot conclude that they are identical by descent. Identity by state analyses are needed to handle this type of data. Unfortunately, the loss of identity by descent information reduces statistical power. This means that, when we use identity by state methods, more relative pairs have to be studied as compared with the numbers needed for identity by descent methods.

> **Key Point:** Although there are many statistical methods for conducting linkage analysis, each method produces two crucial numbers: a statistic that indexes the degree to which a disease and a marker gene are shared among ill family members and a probability value that indicates the probability that the level of sharing observed is due to the play of chance, not linkage.

Another generalization of the sib-pair method uses information from sibs who are not affected with the disease of interest. Thus, instead of studying sibs who are *concordant for disease*, that is, both sibs have the disorder, this method examines pairs constituted of *discordant sibs*, that is, one has the disorder and the other does not. If a DNA marker is linked to a disease, then discordant sibs should share alleles at the marker locus less often then expected by Mendel's laws.

Before moving on to discuss the lod score method of linkage analysis, one other feature of the affected pedigree member method is worth mentioning: we can use the method without knowing the mode of inheritance of the disease. This makes it very appealing for studies of psychiatric disorders. For most of these conditions, we can infer the presence of genes from twin and adoption studies, but mathematical modeling studies have not been able to describe the mode of inheritance.

The Lod Score Method of Linkage Analysis

Like the affected pedigree member method, this second popular approach to linkage analysis computes a statistic, the lod score, which increases in value with evidence for linkage, along with a number indicating the probability that the result was due to chance events. The term "lod" was derived from its method of computation: it is the *lo*garithm of an *od*ds ratio.

The main drawback of the lod score method is that we must specify the mode of genetic transmission. Because segregation studies have not been able to confirm specific modes of inheritance for most psychiatric disorders, some researchers have suggested that psychiatric studies should rely on affected pedigree member methods. However, there is a way around this problem. Dr. David Greenberg showed that if we analyze data several times under different modes of inheritance, the lod score will be the greatest for the model that is closest to the true mode of inheritance. For example, we might choose to examine two dominant models and two recessive models. For each of these we could also vary specific features of the hypothetical disease gene, such as its frequency in the population and the probability that it causes disease. We would then use the model giving the most evidence for linkage as our final result.

To compute a lod score we need a set of families for which we have diagnosed disease status and genotyped DNA markers. We are not limited to affected relatives. All family members are included in the analysis. To derive a lod score from these families, we will need to compute two additional numbers. Each is a "likelihood" computed under a specific assumption about the presence of linkage between disease and marker genes. The first number we compute is the likelihood of observing the pattern of DNA marker and disease co-transmission under the assumption that marker and disease are not linked. Mathematically, this is equivalent to assuming that the probability of crossing over (the recombination fraction) between the disease and marker genes is equal to one half. We use the symbol $L(\frac{1}{2})$ to symbolize the likelihood of no linkage.

The second number needed for the lod score is the largest value possible for the likelihood under all values of the recombination fraction ranging from zero (complete linkage) to one-half (no linkage). A computer program determines this maximum value by computing the likelihood many times. For each computation it assumes a different value for the probability of recombination. These values of the recombination fraction will range from zero to one-half. The recombination fraction is usually represented by the Greek letter θ (theta). It is our estimate of the probability that the disease gene and marker cross over during genetic transmission. You can also think of it as the distance between the disease gene and the DNA marker.

After computing these likelihoods we determine which is the largest. The corresponding value of the recombination fraction is called our "maximum likelihood estimate" (MLE). We symbolize the likelihood as $L(\theta)$. If our estimate of θ is close to zero, that means that the probability of crossing over between disease and marker genes is very low; that is, they are linked. In contrast, if the estimate is close to one-half, we would conclude that the marker and disease genes are distant from one another or on different chromosomes.

As usual, we need a statistic, in this case the lod score, to help us choose between these two possible conclusions. We first compute an odds ratio by dividing $L(\theta)$ by $L(\frac{1}{2})$. For example, if our estimate of θ is one-half, then $L(\theta) = L(\frac{1}{2})$, and the odds ratio is equal to 1, indicating no evidence for linkage. In contrast, if the MLE is less than one-half, then $L(\theta)$ will be greater than $L(\frac{1}{2})$ and the odds ratio will be greater than 1. For example, an odds ratio of 100 would tell us that the odds favoring linkage were 100 times greater than the odds favoring no linkage.

For a variety of reasons that need not concern us, statistical geneticists decided that it was easier to work with the logarithm (to base 10) of the odds ratio rather than with the odds ratio itself. This logarithm is the lod score that you will see reported in scientific journals. Translating a lod score into an odds ratio is easy if you remember the following equation: odds ratio = 10^{lod}. Thus, the odds ratios corresponding to lod scores of 0, 1, 2, 3, and 4 are 1, 10, 100, 1,000, and 10,000, respectively. These increasingly positive lod scores provide increasing evidence for the presence of linkage. When lod scores are negative, they give evidence against linkage. For example, a lod score of 3 indicates that the odds favoring linkage are 1,000 to 1 but a lod score of –3 indicates that the odds against linkage are 1,000 to 1.

For many years, lod scores greater than 3 were considered to be evidence in favor of linkage, while lod scores less than –2 were said to constitute evidence against linkage. Thus, a linkage analysis will support the hypothesis of linkage if the odds favoring linkage are 1,000 to 1 but would reject linkage if the odds against linkage were 100 to 1. These rules worked well for single-gene diseases but were later found to be inadequate for complex diseases. For example, early reports of linkage for both schizophrenia and bipolar disorder were met with much fanfare because studies had found lod scores greater than 3. But when subsequent work failed to confirm these findings, statistical geneticists realized that the rules applied to single-gene diseases could not be applied to complex diseases.

Guidelines for Interpreting Linkage Results

After completing a linkage analysis, we are left with a test statistic and a probability value for each DNA marker tested. As the statistic increases and the probability value decreases, our confidence that we have found linkage increases. For practical purposes, it is essential that we have a decision rule for declaring that a marker is or is not linked to a disease gene. Such rules are needed for asserting the presence of linkage in professional publications. They also serve as guides to determine when more laboratory resources should be allocated to characterize a nearby disease gene that has been detected by linkage analysis.

Thus, before concluding that an apparent linkage is real, we want to be sure that the probability of our being wrong is very low. Although this statement garners widespread support in the scientific community, there is less of a consensus about exactly how low the probability value should be before we can safely conclude that we have detected a disease gene with linkage analysis. If you have even a passing knowledge of statistics, you may recall that the 5 percent probability level is, by convention, widely accepted as the threshold for believing that an observation is not due to chance. Thus, for most statistical applications, if the probability value is lower than 5 percent we will conclude that chance did not produce our results.

But there are several reasons why the 5 percent level is not appropriate for genetic linkage analysis. Most importantly, a linkage analysis consists not of a single statistical test, but of many tests, one for each DNA marker tested. For example, we might use 400 markers for our initial scan of the genome and then an additional 100 to follow up on regions implicated by the initial scan. Statisticians have shown that we must adjust the 5 percent probability threshold when we perform many statistical tests. This consideration, along with other arcane statistical genetic issues, has led to the concept of the genomewide significance level—the probability threshold that we should use for declaring linkage after testing the many DNA markers used for a genome scan.

Drs. Eric Lander and Leonid Kruglyak proposed guidelines for genomewide significance levels that have gained acceptance among many scientists. They suggest that we adopt three levels of confidence when discussing linkage results. *Suggestive linkage* refers to statistical evidence that we would expect to find one time by chance during a genome scan. For the sib-pair method, we can assert suggestive linkage if the probability value is less than .0007. For the lod score method, the value is .0017. *Significant linkage* refers to evidence we would expect to find .05 times by chance during a genome scan. For the sib-pair method, we can assert suggestive linkage if the probability value is less than .00002. For the lod score method, the value is .000049.

Despite the stringency of these probability levels, to use the term *confirmed linkage*, Drs. Lander and Kruglyak's guidelines require that a significant linkage has been found in an initial genome scan and has subsequently been confirmed in an independent sample. This second step is necessary because, if only one study detects linkage, we cannot be sure if that might have been due to unusual features of the study design or the sample studied.

Drs. Lander and Kruglyak's guidelines provide a handy index for evaluating linkage results reported in scientific journals or the news media. For example, a hypothetical news report might shout the title "Schizophrenia Gene Found!" Perhaps the news article quotes the title of the paper as "Report of Potential Linkage between Schizophrenia and Chromosome 10." You should immediately wonder what "potential" means. A look at the article might show you that the probability value for the putative schizophrenia linkage was only .001, much less than the guidelines require for us to conclude that linkage truly exists.

Examples of Linkage Analysis

Linkage studies in psychiatric disorders have been fraught with problems. Over the past 30 years, researchers have reported positive linkage studies for many psychiatric disorders, only to have their findings refuted by subsequent studies. This pattern occurred in scientific reports linking chromosome 15 to learning disability, chromosome 5 to schizophrenia, and chromosomes 11 and X to bipolar disorder. However, the tide may be turning. Recent linkage analysis studies have replicated initial reports of positive linkage to chromosome 6 markers in families with schizophrenia. Although there are several negative studies, the evidence implicating the short arm of chromosome 6 is the strongest to date for schizophrenia. Unfortunately, the region of interest is so large (about 30 million base-pairs), it is not feasible to use laboratory methods to pinpoint the disease gene. Typically, actually finding the gene requires linkage methods to narrow the region of interest to less than 2 million base-pairs.

One exceptional success for psychiatric linkage studies is seen in the study of Alzheimer disease, where several genes have been discovered. For example, Dr. Gerard Schellenberg and colleagues first reported a positive genetic linkage on chromosome 14 for early-onset familial Alzheimer disease (FAD). Table 5.1 shows the lod scores for linkage between FAD and chromosome 14 markers. Each lod score corresponds to a DNA marker indicated by the row header and an estimated recombination fraction indicated by the column header. For example, the lod score of –10.34 in the first row and column is for marker TCRD and a recombination fraction of .001. This very negative lod score clearly suggests that FAD is not closely linked to TCRD. In fact, because all of the lod scores in row 1 are negative, we can conclude that there is not an FAD gene in the vicinity of the marker.

In contrast, examine the lod scores for DNA marker D14S53. A maximum lod score of 7.12 was obtained at recombination fraction of .05. This suggested to Dr. Schellenberg that the FAD gene might be close to D14S53. The lod scores were even higher for D14S43, suggesting that the region around that marker harbored an FAD disease gene. In fact, as we will discuss later, when Dr. Schellenberg and colleagues

TABLE 5.1. Lod Scores for Linkage of Alzheimer Disease to DNA Markers on Chromosome 14

DNA marker	Recombination fraction						
	0.001	0.05	0.10	0.15	0.20	0.30	0.40
TCRD	–10.34	–4.52	–2.84	–1.86	–1.21	–0.44	–0.09
D14S47	–5.29	–0.87	–0.01	0.35	0.48	0.39	0.15
D14S52	2.02	4.59	4.56	4.19	3.64	2.25	0.08
D14S43	**8.91**	**8.40**	**7.67**	**6.79**	**5.79**	**3.55**	**1.33**
D14S53	4.24	7.12	6.88	6.19	5.28	3.10	0.99
D14S55	–1.32	0.43	0.66	0.70	0.64	0.43	0.19
D14S48	–10.96	–2.56	–0.93	–0.15	0.25	0.41	0.13
AACT	–2.35	0.06	0.52	0.68	0.69	0.46	0.16
PI	–9.72	–2.52	–0.69	0.55	0.61	0.61	0.24
D14S1	–17.70	–5.10	–2.08	–0.59	0.20	0.69	0.47

examined this region further, they unequivocally established that a gene on chromosome 14 caused Alzheimer disease in the families they had studied.

ASSOCIATION STUDIES

Linkage analysis has been extremely successful for diseases with well-defined modes of inheritance. But, with the exception of Alzheimer disease, it has not yet gleaned genes for psychiatric disorders. Because of this, some investigators have turned to association studies and related techniques.

Population-Based Association Studies

A scientist originally developed the population-based association study to study specific genes believed, for theoretical reasons, to be involved in the etiology of a disorder. Such genes are called "candidate genes" to indicate that they are suitable candidates for study. For example, because the effects of antipsychotic medications are believed to be mediated through their impact on D2 dopamine receptors in the brain, the gene that encodes the D2 receptor has been considered a candidate gene for schizophrenia.

The method of association is very easy to understand. Assume, for example, that there are two versions of the D2 receptor. We will call these versions D2-1 and D2-2. To study these variants in schizophrenia, we would collect DNA samples from a sample of schizophrenic patients and from a sample of controls. After genotyping the samples, we could compare the two groups to determine if one allele was more frequently seen among schizophrenic patients. If, for example, D2-2 was more common among the patients, that would suggest that the D2-2 variant was involved in the etiology of schizophrenia. We write "suggest" because there are several reasons why that conclusion might be wrong.

First, to meaningfully compare gene frequencies between patients and controls, we must be certain that the two groups are well matched for ethnic background. Population geneticists have shown that gene variants are not evenly distributed among ethnic groups. For example, they have shown that the 7-repeat variant of the D4 dopamine gene is more common among Caucasian than Chinese people. Clearly, a comparison of Caucasian patients with Chinese controls would be meaningless.

The effects of ethnicity can also be more subtle than in this extreme situation. There is, for example, no guarantee that gene variants are similar between British and Italian people or even between northern and southern Italians. Thus, population-based association studies are most meaningful when patients and controls come from a very well defined population. *Population isolates* are especially useful: these are groups of people who are very ethnically homogeneous because they have been isolated from the rest of the world for some time. Such populations are usually found on islands, for example, Iceland, or in mountainous regions, for example, the Basques in the Pyrenees, that are not easily accessible.

Second, another weak inferential link when reasoning from association studies is the fact that a positive association finding for a specific gene could occur if that gene was very close to the true disease gene. But as we shall see, this weakness of the association method is also a hidden strength due to a biological condition called "linkage disequilibrium." As you know from our discussion of crossing over, the genes on a chromosome are reshuffled during genetic transmission. You also know that if two genes are located very close to one another on a chromosome, then they will rarely be separated by crossing over and will usually be transmitted together. Thus, due to close linkage, the alleles at two genetic loci will tend to be transmitted together. We write "tend to" because eventually crossing over will separate them.

When genes are far apart, they are quickly reshuffled. But when they are very close together, the reshuffling can take many thousands of years. When genes are so close that they rarely are separated by crossing over, we say they are in "linkage disequilibrium." We will illustrate the effects of linkage disequilibrium with the following hypothetical example. Suppose that the D2 gene is very close to an unknown schizophrenia disease gene we will call X. Many years ago, X mutated from the harmless X-1 form to the X-2 form, which increased susceptibility to schizophrenia. The person in whom this mutation occurred happened by chance to have the D2-2 variant of the D2 gene on the same chromosome as the X-2 allele. Because the D2 and X genes are very closely linked to one another, when X-2 is transmitted to a child, D2-2 is usually transmitted as well, although, rarely, they are separated by crossing over.

Now, many hundreds of years later, a scientist genotypes the D2 gene in schizophrenic patients and ethnically matched controls. She finds that D2-2 is more common among the schizophrenic patients and concludes that mutations in the D2 gene cause schizophrenia. But she is wrong. It is the X gene that causes schizophrenia. D2-2 is associated with the disease because it is in linkage disequilibrium with X-2.

If you understand why the scientist made an inferential error, you will also understand how we can use linkage disequilibrium to our advantage. Because of linkage disequilibrium, we do not need a candidate gene to use the association method. We can use any DNA marker. In fact, Dr. Neil Risch has suggested that by examining many DNA markers very closely spaced along the chromosomes, we can screen the entire genome using the method of association. The markers must be very closely spaced because linkage disequilibrium only occurs over very small segments of DNA. As of this writing, a full genome scan association study is not possible because we do not have enough closely spaced markers. But, given the pace of DNA marker development, such studies should be feasible in the near future.

If you wish to fully grasp the differences between linkage and association studies, it is essential that you understand the difference between the terms "linkage" and "linkage disequilibrium." We say that a marker and a disease gene are linked if they are so close to one another that the probability of them being separated during crossing over is less than the probability of them being transmitted together. We say that a marker and disease gene are in linkage disequilibrium when they are so very, very close to one another that the reshuffling of genes that occurs over many generations has completely separated the mutant version of the disease gene from the version of the marker that happened to be alongside it when the original mutation occurred.

When a gene and a marker are linked, members of the same family who are ill will usually also carry the same version of a closely linked genetic marker. But the version of the marker will vary from family to family. For example, suppose we find linkage between schizophrenia and a marker on chromosome 10. In one family, all of the schizophrenic siblings may have version A of the marker. In another family, the schizophrenic siblings may all have version B. The marker version differs between families because in the first family the parent carrying the schizophrenia gene happened to have marker version A. In the second family, the parent carrying the schizophrenia gene happened to have marker version B.

When a gene and a marker are in linkage disequilibrium, ill members from different families will tend to have the same version of the genetic marker. So if version A of the marker was next to the disease gene when the original mutation occurred, most people with schizophrenia will have version A of the marker allele.

> **Key Point:** A simple way to avoid confusing "linkage" and "linkage disequilibrium" is to remember two key points:

1. Linkage leads to ill members of the same family having the same version of the marker, whereas linkage disequilibrium leads to ill members of the same or different families having the same version of the marker.

2. Because linkage disequilibrium occurs over very short stretches of DNA, we can detect its existence only if our DNA marker is very close to the gene. In contrast, we can detect linkage over greater genetic distances.

The study of the apolipoprotein-E (APOE) gene in Alzheimer disease provides a successful example of a population-based association study. Dr. Allen Roses and colleagues first reported that, among Alzheimer patients the frequency of the APOE ε4 allele was significantly higher than that found in controls (36 percent vs. 16 percent). Since then, many studies have confirmed this association.

In an Alzheimer disease patient registry based in the largest health maintenance organization in the Seattle area, one of the authors (DT) working with Drs. Walter Kukull and Eric Larson also found this association. As the top part of Table 5.2 shows, the ε4/ε3 and ε4/ε4 genotypes were more common among Alzheimer patients compared with controls. The bottom part of the table shows that the ε4 allele was almost three times more frequent among Alzheimer patients.

Although these data along with over 100 other studies show that the ε4 allele of the APOE gene is associated with Alzheimer disease, they also show that it is not a necessary cause of the disease. We see this in the first three rows of the first column of Table 5.2, which shows that 42 percent of Alzheimer disease cases do not carry the ε4 allele. This suggests that other factors (either genetic or environmental) contribute to the development of Alzheimer disease in these people. In addition, there were 80 controls in their 80s with an ε4 allele who did not have dementia. This suggests that the ε4 allele is not a sufficient cause of Alzheimer disease; some other cause is needed for the disease to occur.

The association studies of Alzheimer disease are especially convincing because linkage analysis has demonstrated suggestive linkage between the disease and APOE using linkage analysis methodology. Moreover, biological features of APOE make it a theoretically reasonable candidate gene for Alzheimer disease. The gene encodes APOE, a cholesterol-carrying protein that binds tightly to the senile plaques that are found in the brains of Alzheimer patients at autopsy. Scientists are now studying how the differences in the protein's binding capacity might lead to the disease.

TABLE 5.2. APOE Genotypes and Allele Frequencies in the Community Sample Cases and Controls

	Community sample Alzheimer disease cases $n = 234$ (%)	Community sample controls $n = 304$ (%)
	Genotypes	
ε2/ε2	0	4 (1.3)
ε3/ε2	8 (3.4)	38 (12.5)
ε3/ε3	90 (38.5)	182 (59.9)
ε4/ε2	10 (4.3)	15 (4.9)
ε4/ε3	96 (41.0)	63 (20.7)
ε4/ε4	30 (12.8)	2 (0.7)
	Allele frequencies (95% C.I.)	
ε2	0.04 (0.02–0.06)	0.10 (0.08–0.12)
ε3	0.60 (0.56–0.65)	0.76 (0.73–0.80)
ε4	**0.36** (0.31–0.40)	**0.13** (0.11–0.16)

Note. Adapted from Tsuang, D., Kukull, W., Sheppard, L., Barnhart, R., Peksind, E., Edland, S., Schellenberg, G., Raskind, M., & Larson, E. B. (1996). Impact of sample selection on APOE ε4 allele frequency: A comparison of two Alzheimer's disease samples. *Journal of the American Geriatric Society, 44,* 704–707. Copyright 1996 by Lippincott Williams & Wilkins. Adapted with permission.

Family-Based Association Studies

Despite the success of population-based association studies for Alzheimer and other diseases, the interpretation of such studies is often clouded by potential ethnic differences between patient and control groups. To address this problem, statistical geneticists developed tests of linkage disequilibrium that use the parents or siblings of ill individuals as controls.

For example, the transmission test for linkage disequilibrium (TDT) uses families having at least one affected offspring and two parents who provide a DNA sample. We do not need to know the parents' diagnoses but we must have their DNA. As you know from Mendel's laws, each parent transmits only one allele of each gene to the ill child. To compute the TDT test, we compare the alleles transmitted by parents to those that were not transmitted. The nontransmitted alleles serve as the control group for the transmitted alleles. Because both the transmitted and the nontransmitted alleles come from the same parent, they are perfectly matched for ethnicity.

Consider the following table:

Nontransmitted alleles		D2-1	D2-2
Transmitted alleles	D2-1	25	5
	D2-2	65	5

The table presents hypothetical data from 50 families. There are 100 subjects in the table because each family contributes two parents. Each number in the table tells us how many parents had each possible pair of transmitted and nontransmitted alleles. For example, the number 5 in the lower right corner tells us that five parents transmitted a D2-2 allele to the ill child but for these five parents the nontransmitted allele was also D2-2. These parents are called "homozygous for the D2 gene" because they have two identical alleles of that gene. The table also shows that 25 additional parents are homozygous because they had two copies of the D2-1 gene. Homozygous parents cannot provide information about gene–disease associations because, by definition, the allele they transmit must be the same as the one they do not transmit.

In contrast, the heterozygous parents provide us with much useful information. We say a person is "heterozygous for a gene" if he or she carries two different versions of the gene. There are 70 heterozygous parents in the table. Sixty-five of these transmitted the D2-2 allele and did not transmit the D2-1 allele. Only 5 parents transmitted the D2-1 allele and did not transmit the D2-2 allele. Thus, these data suggest that the D2-2 alleles are preferentially transmitted to the affected offspring.

In general, the TDT compares the number of times heterozygous parents transmit the associated marker to affected offspring with the number of times they transmit the other marker. If these probabilities differ from what is expected by chance, then we can conclude that linkage disequilibrium exists, that is, that the gene is associated with the disease.

Although the TDT test and other family-based association methods solve the problem of ethnic matching, they still require that the gene used in the analysis is either the disease gene or one very close to the disease gene. This is in contrast with the linkage method which can detect linkage over relatively large genetic distances. Thus, with linkage analysis it is currently possible to "scan the genome," which is a shorthand way of saying that if we use many markers, we can test for linkage in all chromosomal locations. In contrast, at this time it is not possible to completely scan the genome using the method of association. Thus, for such a study to succeed we need to know where to find the putative gene. So how do we know where to look?

The typical approach to this problem is to make some educated guesses. When we make such a guess we are specifying a candidate gene. Once we have a candidate, we proceed with the association study. Ideally a candidate gene should have a known pathophysiologic significance in the disorder of interest. For example, Alzheimer disease leaves a clear pathophysiologic signature on the brain (senile plaques containing ß-amyloid) Since the production of ß-amyloid requires the amyloid precursor protein (APP), the APP gene was a logical candidate gene for Alzheimer disease. Studies of the APP gene among some families with Alzheimer disease patients found unequivocal genetic changes or mutations that are only found in affected individuals.

Unlike Alzheimer disease, most psychiatric disorders do not have a known pathophysiology that points to an obvious candidate gene. For example, although schizophrenia is undoubtedly a disease of the brain, the pathophysiologic details have eluded careful investigation. There are many thousands of genes that *might* be relevant to schizophrenia, but none of these are credible candidate genes in the sense that the APP gene was a credible candidate for Alzheimer disease. For example, we know that neurotransmitter systems are dysregulated in many psychiatric disorders. We also know the locations of various neurotransmitter genes and segments of genes encoding monoamine oxidase, dopamine-beta-hydroxylase, tyrosine hydroxylase, and dopamine receptor genes have been screened for mutations and genetic variations. Unfortunately, none of these genes have consistently yielded differences between schizophrenic patients and normal controls.

Psychiatric geneticists have tried to capitalize on plausible links between such genes and psychiatric illness but not without controversy. The failure of association studies to produce consistently reproducible results supports Dr. Raymond Crowe's contention that "candidate genes in psychiatry are lottery tickets." As Dr. Crowe discussed, there are approximately 30,000 genes expressed in the human brain. Any of these could be a "candidate" for psychiatric disease, yet none are well justified to the same degree that the APP gene was a credible candidate for Alzheimer disease. As a result, the a priori probability is low that any one of these is associated with a specific disease.

> **Key Point:** The results of family-based association studies are likely to be less biased than those of case–control studies unless the latter type of study selects cases and controls from an ethnically homogeneous population.

Because of the problems discussed above, association studies must be used and interpreted with caution. Dr. Kenneth Kidd suggested that consistent replication would be the best evidence for a true association. However, he also cautioned that to be a true replication, a subsequent study should use methods that are similar if not identical to the methods of the original study. This consistency is evident in the association between the APOE ε4 allele and Alzheimer disease, where over 100 studies have replicated this finding.

THE SEARCH FOR DISEASE MECHANISMS

Finding Mutations That Cause Disease

Once a linkage analysis maps a DNA marker within a few million base-pairs of the putative gene, the search for the gene can begin. Since many genes are likely present within that region, more detailed analyses are necessary to identify the affected gene. In general, DNA from this region is studied intensively. The first step is to saturate the region with many closely spaced DNA markers. This process narrows down the size of the region that contains the gene.

Next, a map of nearby genes can be constructed and DNA fragments can be screened for variations. Furthermore, by comparing the putative region with established maps of genes known to exist in that region, individual candidate genes can be examined. Eventually, candidate genes can be sequenced in both affected and unaffected individuals. "To sequence a gene" means to determine the exact order of the base-pairs in that gene.

If, for a specific candidate gene, affected individuals consistently show a base-pair sequence that differs from that found among unaffected individuals, we can conclude that a disease gene has been discovered. Although this is a crucial step, it is only the beginning of another process: understanding the chain of events whereby the gene and environmental events lead to disease. For example, using the sequence of the abnormal gene, researchers can determine how the mutation affects the structure of the protein that the gene encodes. Further study of the protein can eventually provide the biochemical basis of the disease.

The study of Alzheimer disease provides a good example of how genes are discovered. Three years after Dr. Gerard Schellenberg detected linkage for an Alzheimer gene on chromosome 14, Harvard University researchers identified this gene. The gene, called presenilin 1, was sequenced and determined to be a protein that traversed cell membranes. Since then over 43 different pathogenic mutations in presenilin 1 have been found in over 60 unrelated Alzheimer disease families.

Subsequently, Dr. Schellenberg's group found a very similar gene, presenilin 2, on chromosome 1. This gene was linked to early-onset Alzheimer disease in an ethnically distinct subgroup of families (the Volga Germans). In families linked to presenilin 1 or presenilin 2, mutations were found only among the family members having Alzheimer disease. This strongly suggested that mutations in presenilin 2 caused Alzheimer disease in these families.

The exact mechanism by which the presenilin genes cause Alzheimer disease is unknown but their discovery has opened up new avenues for both human and animal research investigating the pathogenesis of the disorder. As the mechanism of disease becomes clear, researchers will be able to develop new treatments that target either the mutant gene or its protein product. Although currently difficult to implement, we will discuss this and other treatment alternatives in Chapter 7.

Types of Mutations

A *mutation* is any permanent change in the DNA sequence of a gene. These genetic aberrations can be caused by environmental toxins or by errors during *meiosis,* the process whereby chromosomes are duplicated in preparation for genetic transmission. These changes lead to a variant protein, which may result in disease.

In some cases, these mutational events will cut the DNA strand in two places, freeing a small piece of DNA from two larger pieces of the chromosome. Although the cell can repair broken DNA, the repair is not always 100 percent correct. If the DNA mechanic connects the two larger pieces, the resulting chromosome has a *deletion mutation*. In such a case, a segment of DNA is permanently lost. The loss of DNA within a gene means that part of the genetic code is missing. Hence, the gene cannot produce the correct protein. It is also possible that the chromosomal segment deleted from one chromosome will be tacked on to the end of another to produce a *translocation mutation*. Translocations are not always clinically relevant because in many cases genes are simply transferred from one chromosome to another. But they can cause problems if one of the breakpoints in the chromosome occurs in the middle of a gene.

Another possibility is that the small piece of DNA reproduces itself and then, during the repair process, is inserted twice into the original chromosome. This type of error is known as a *duplication mutation*. If the DNA mechanic cannot find the missing small piece of DNA, it may use another errant piece of DNA instead. This creates an *insertion muta-tion*. Sometimes the DNA mechanic finds the correct piece of DNA but inserts it in reverse order. This creates an *inversion mutation*..

The ease with which mutations are detected depends, in part, on how large the affected portion of the chromosome is. The larger the mutated DNA segment, the easier it is to find. But not all mutations are large and even very small ones can have devastating effects. One of the major challenges for molecular genetics is to find the minute mutations known as *point mutations*, which involve a single base-pair within the gene's DNA sequence. This single base-pair may be deleted or it may be replaced by another base-pair.

One type of point mutation is the *nonsense mutation* in which a base-pair sequence that signals further protein construction changes to one signaling the end of protein construction. In this case, the genetic code becomes so garbled that no protein can be produced. Alterna-tively, base-pair changes may lead to *missense mutations*. In this case, protein construction is not stopped; instead, the wrong protein is pro-duced.

Trinucleotide repeat mutations are a separate class of mutations. They occur when a triplet sequence of base-pairs is repeated several times within a gene. For example, these mutations have been seen in Huntington disease, a neurodegenerative condition characterized by abnormal motor movements, psychiatric symptoms, and cognitive im-pairments. Typically, in unaffected individuals, the base-pair sequence CAG is repeated 18 times or less within the gene known to cause Hun-tington disease; in Huntington disease patients, at least one of their Huntington disease genes has 39 or more CAG repeat sequences. This results in a longer protein, whose function is not yet known.

Trinucleotide repeat mutations have intrigued psychiatric geneti-cists because they lead to unusual clinical features that have been seen in psychiatric conditions. These mutations lead to a decreasing age at onset and an increasing severity of illness in successive generations of affected family members. We call this phenomenon "genetic anticipa-tion" because milder symptoms in parents appear to anticipate the more severe condition that will afflict their offspring.

The discovery of trinucleotide repeats provided a biological expla-nation for anticipation: the number of repeats may increase during for-mation of an egg or sperm. The resulting increase in repeat size leads to a larger mutation, one that has more deleterious effects, including an earlier onset and increased severity. For example, Huntington dis-ease patients with a large number of repeats (> 60) typically develop symptoms before age 20, whereas a much later onset is common for pa-tients with fewer repeats. Notably, some researchers have observed the clinical features of genetic anticipation in families with bipolar affective disorder and schizophrenia. Although this suggests that trinucleotide repeats may cause these disorders, attempts to confirm this thesis have not been consistently successful.

Many laboratory methods are used to search for mutations. One example is the method of *repeat expansion detection*, which determines if trinucleotide repeats occur anywhere in the genome. Although this method is very useful for establishing the presence of trinucleotide repeats, it cannot determine where the repeats occur.

Another approach, described, by Drs. Janet Sobell and Stephen Sommer, is the "VAPSE-based case–control association study." A VAPSE is a DNA sequence variation affecting protein structure or expression. We find VAPSEs with DNA sequencing, the direct examination of the base-pair sequence that forms the DNA. Any modified sequence that changes the DNA blueprint is a VAPSE. By definition, VAPSEs occur only in regions of the genome that code for proteins or that regulate biological processes—junk DNA cannot constitute a VAPSE.

There are five phases of a VAPSE study: (1) Select one or more candidate genes, that is, genes that can theoretically be implicated in the disorder under study; (2) use a subset of patients to search for VAPSEs; (3) if you find a VAPSE, use a larger group of affected and unaffected people to see if the disease is associated with the VAPSE; (4) replicate the observed association; and (5) determine if the VAPSE and the disease are linked using linkage analyses in families that exhibit the VAPSE.

Theoretically, we could screen the entire genome for VAPSEs and potentially find all the genes responsible for any complex disorder. Unfortunately, this tactic is not currently feasible because it is too expensive and time-consuming. The problem is too many gene variants that probably have no functional significance. They might alter a protein, but not sufficiently so as to cause diseases. That is why we must focus on candidate genes to use this approach to mutation detection.

Cytogenetic Abnormalities and Psychiatric Disorders

Linkage and association studies are typically used to discover genes when the mutations that cause disease are too small to be detected by the direct examination of chromosomes known as *cytogenetics*. When stained with dyes and examined under a microscope, each of our 23 pairs of chromosomes can be distinguished from one another. Figure 5.5 shows how the chromosomes differ not only in size but also in the pattern of bands produced by staining. We know that the chromosomes in Figure 5.5 came from a female because there are two X chromosomes.

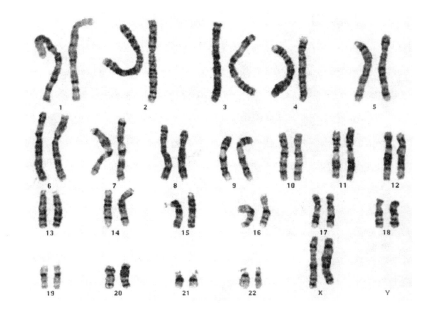

FIGURE 5.5. A normal female karyotype. Courtesy of Christine Disteche, PhD, Cytogenetics Laboratory, University of Washington, Seattle, Washington.

Figure 5.6 is a schematic representation of the chromosomes with their unique bands. The physical features of chromosomes provide us with several landmarks to use when discussing the location of genes. The place where the chromosomes appear to be tied together is the *centromere*, which divides the chromosome into two arms. By convention, the short arm is called "p" and the long arm "q." Thus, when we say that a schizophrenia gene was detected on chromosome 6p, we mean that the DNA markers that showed linkage were on the short arm of the sixth chromosome. Each arm of a chromosome is further divided into regions delimited by specific landmarks, which are distinct structural features observable under a microscope. Then the regions are subdivided into bands. The bands can be easily distinguished from an adjacent part in the chromosome by the intensity of staining (see Figure 5.6).

Figure 5.7 shows the cytogenetic subdivisions of chromosome 6. As you can see, we number the bands and regions from the centromere outward. Each digit is referred to separately. For example, the band 6p12 refers to the p arm of chromosome 6, region 1 and band 2. It is pronounced as "six-p one-two." It is important to realize that bands do not correspond to genes. In fact, they are very large areas likely to include hundreds of genes and DNA markers. As an example, Figure 5.7 shows only a few of the many markers that are located on 6p.

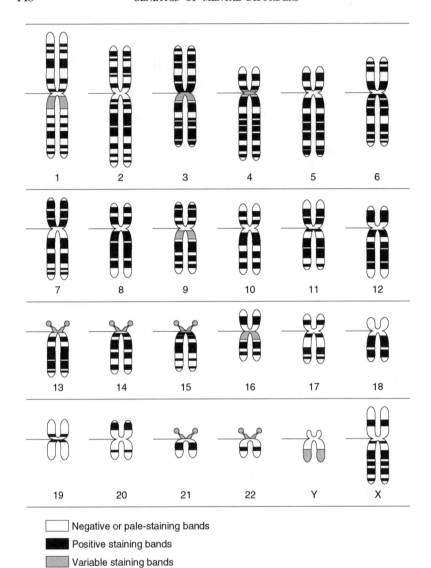

1	2	3	4	5	6
7	8	9	10	11	12
13	14	15	16	17	18
19	20	21	22	Y	X

☐ Negative or pale-staining bands
■ Positive staining bands
▨ Variable staining bands

FIGURE 5.6. Representation of the human genome, consisting of 22 pairs of autosomes and 1 pair of sex chromosomes.

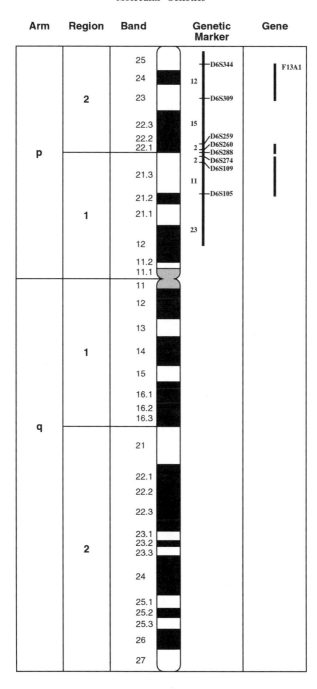

FIGURE 5.7. Schematic representation of chromosome 6, with delineation of specific arm, region, sample bands, genetic markers, and genes.

In addition to providing a useful language for describing the structure of chromosomes, cytogenetic methods also allow us to detect relatively large changes in chromosomal structure. We describe cytogenetic abnormalities as "relatively large" because we can detect them with a microscopic examination of the chromosomes. For example, different kinds of cytogenetic stains allow scientists to identify missing, extra, or grossly aberrant chromosomes. In medical genetics, a routine cytogenetic study would screen for obvious abnormalities in chromosomal number, rearrangement, and shape.

One of the most common chromosomal abnormalities is the *trisomy*, the existence of three copies of the same chromosome, instead of the usual two copies. For example, patients with Down syndrome have an extra chromosome 21. Trisomies occur during the process of egg or sperm formation when chromosomal pairs separate. A Normal egg or sperm should have only one chromosome. Sometimes if proper separation does not occur, some egg or sperm receive two chromosomes while others receive no chromosomes. If the egg containing two chromosomes is fertilized, the resulting embryo would have three copies of the chromosome. Trisomies usually result in spontaneous abortions but some may result in viable births. Another example is Kleinfelter syndrome, which affects men who have an extra X chromosome (i.e., they have three sex chromosomes: XXY instead of XY).

Other types of cytogenetic abnormalities involve rearrangements of chromosomal material. These include deletions and translocations. The term *deletions* refers to a missing segment of a chromosome. An example is cri du chat syndrome. The English translation of the French "cri du chat" is "cry of the cat." This unusual name reflects a key clinical feature: the cry of a newborn having the syndrome sounds like that of a cat. People with cri du chat syndrome are missing part of the tip of chromosome 5. *Translocations* occur when chromosomes break apart and are rejoined into new combinations. If no genes are lost then the person may be normal. But if the rearrangement results in extra or missing genes, abnormalities may result.

By now you must be wondering if cytogenetic studies have discovered chromosomal abnormalities that lead to psychiatric disorders. The answer is both yes and no. Typically, when psychiatric patients have been screened with cytogenetic methods, some abnormalities have been found but only in a minority of patients. For example, several cytogenetic abnormalities have been seen in schizophrenic patients, but these occur in less than 1 percent of patients.

Although cytogenetic abnormalities are rare among psychiatric patients, they may still facilitate the discovery of disease genes. This possibility is seen in the case of Duchenne muscular dystrophy. Although most cases of this disease show no cytogenetic abnormalities, one boy with Duchenne muscular dystrophy had a small deletion on the X chromosome. This finding eventually led to identification of the gene causing Duchenne muscular dystrophy. Thus, unusual cases can provide key information about the location of disease genes. Although the amount of DNA implicated by a cytogenetic abnormality can be large, it does allow investigators to narrow their search for pathogenic genes from the entire genome to the region implicated by the cytogenetic finding.

One example from psychiatry was Dr. Ann Bassett's report of a man and his nephew who both had schizophrenia-like symptoms and multiple physical anomalies. Both of these people had an extra copy of segments from the long arm of chromosome 5. These cytogenetic findings generated much excitement. Following this lead, several investigators performed linkage studies using DNA markers in this region. Although these studies have not yet confirmed the presence of a schizophrenia gene on chromosome 5, the search for cytogenetic abnormalities may yet prove worthwhile.

Dr. Bassett recommends that clinicians continue to look for cytogenetic abnormalities. Although it would not be sensible to routinely screen for these problems, you should be alert for cases with unusual clinical features that present with mental handicaps or physical anomalies such as unusual facial features or the presence of multiple organ abnormalities.

The advent of sophisticated cytogenetic techniques that can define smaller chromosomal regions may also help in the search for genes associated with psychiatric disorders. An example of this new technology includes fluorescent *in situ* hybridization, or FISH. FISH capitalizes on the fact that DNA consists of two complementary strands connected by base-pairs. When the DNA from a patient's chromosome is heated, it denatures, or "unzips," so that the two strands separate. When the DNA mixture is cooled, each strand will naturally seek to connect, or "hybridize," with its partner.

To use this feature of DNA, scientists unzip a chromosome and mix the strands into a cocktail containing an artificial segment of DNA that codes for a specific gene known to be on the chromosome that has been mixed into the cocktail. This piece of DNA is colored with a fluorescent dye. When the cocktail is cooled, the colored DNA will hybridize with the patient's DNA if the patient's DNA contains the sequence encoded by the colored DNA. If that gene does not exist in the patient's DNA, then the colored DNA will not hybridize. So, after the cocktail has cooled sufficiently, we examine the patient's DNA. If any of the strands are connected to the colored, artificial DNA, we know that the gene exists on the patient's chromosome. Otherwise, we can conclude that the gene does not exist, that is, that the patient has a small deletion. The main advantage of FISH is its ability to detect the very small chromosomal deletions that are not evident from microscopic examination.

> **Key Point:** Most cases of mental illness cannot be attributed to cytogenetic abnormalities. Nevertheless, because some of these abnormalities lead to psychopathology, understanding the nature and location of these abnormalities can provide insights into the rough location of the genes responsible for the majority of cases of mental illness.

Microdeletion syndromes are an example of chromosomal deletions that can be detected by FISH. They involve a deletion of consecutive genes and are therefore also known as contiguous gene syndromes. Because microdeletion syndromes affect multiple genes, they usually cause multiple abnormalities. One example, velo-cardio-facial syndrome (VCFS), is relevant to psychiatric genetics. In VCFS patients, deletions of chromosome 22q cause learning disabilities, cleft palate, pharyngeal hypotonia, and/or cardiac anomalies. Dr. Ann Pulver and colleagues examined patients diagnosed with VCFS along with their relatives. Interestingly, they found a higher rate of psychosis compared to the general population, and suggested that there may be a gene associated with schizophrenia on chromosome 22q. This region is known to contain the catechol-O-methyltransferase (COMT) gene. Moreover, several linkage studies of this region reported data consistent with the presence of a schizophrenia gene in the region. These findings, however, are not strong enough for us to conclude that linkage has been confirmed. Nevertheless, 22q is currently considered as a strong candidate region for schizophrenia.

Animal Models of Human Disorders

At first blush, it seems unlikely that studies of other animals could tell us anything about the genetic mechanisms of human mental illness. After all, humans are complex creatures; their psychological, emotional, and social manifestations would seem far removed from the experiences of other animals. Is it possible that an experiment with rats could tell us much about why humans become mentally ill?

To understand why the answer to this question is "yes" you need to understand the concept of *homologous structures*. In biology, anatomical structures in different animals are homologous if they are similar in structure and have similar evolutionary origins, even though they may serve different functions. A simple example is the human hand and that of a chimpanzee or even the flippers of a seal. As this simple anatomical example shows, there can be different degrees of homology between different types of animals.

Because homologies are also found at the chromosomal and gene level, scientists have found that many human genes are homologous to genes found in the genomes of other animals. Surprisingly, about 85 percent of genes found in mice are also found in humans. So, at the genetic level, the answer to the question "Are you a man or a mouse?" is not so simple.

We also know that some animal behaviors provide models of human mental disorders. In this usage, the term "model" means that the animal behaviors are similar but not identical to some of the signs of the human disorder. For example, in mice we can create a syndrome of "learned helplessness" that has been used as a model of depression. Other mice, that show high levels of hyperactivity, are used as models of attention-deficit hyperactivity disorder. Moreover, because mice can become dependent on alcohol and drugs, they can provide models of substance dependence.

In genetic studies, two types of animal models have been used extensively: the transgenic mouse and the knockout mouse. The *transgenic mouse* is a mouse whose genome has been altered by the insertion of a gene from another species. Scientists create these mice to study mutations that cause an increase in some biological activity that leads to disease. One example from medical genetics is the study of *oncogenes*, genes that cause cancer. Abnormal oncogenes cause accelerated cell division. To create a transgenic mouse, DNA containing the human cancer mutation is injected into the nucleus of a fertilized mouse egg. As a result, the human DNA becomes part of the mouse genome and is passed down to its offspring. Thus, researchers can quickly produce a large number of mice with the human oncogene. Examining the genes' effects on cancer initiation and growth in the mouse leads to insights about the mechanism of disease in humans. These insights can lead to new treatments which can be tested on the mice and, if successful, eventually used in humans.

The *knockout mouse* allows us to study the effects of mutations that stop a gene from functioning. Instead of injecting a new gene into the mouse genome as is done for the transgenic mouse, we create a knockout mouse by removing both copies of a gene from the mouse's genome. This technique allows the development of genetically engineered animals who lack the gene and therefore cannot produce a specific protein. By studying these mice we learn about the effects of mutations that prevent normal gene functioning.

For example, Dr. Marc Caron described a knockout mouse who was missing the dopamine transporter gene. *Dopamine* is a neurotransmitter that is sent from one brain cell to another during brain activity. After a dopamine signal is sent from one cell to another, the dopamine transporter quickly removes dopamine from the space between the cells to signal the end of the message. For normal mice, the removal of dopamine occurs in about 1 second. But when the dopamine transporter has been "knocked out," dopamine lingers for about 100 seconds. Interestingly, this knockout mouse exhibits hyperactivity suggesting that the dopamine transporter plays an important role in level of motor activity. Moreover, using association study methods, Dr. Edwin Cook reported an association between alleles of the dopamine transporter gene and attention-deficit hyperactivity disorder in humans.

Studies of insulin-dependent juvenile-onset diabetes illustrate the potential of animal models to find clinically relevant genes. Studies of mice identified a dozen genes that each made a partial contribution to the disorder. The discovery of these mouse diabetes genes stimulated human research that detected five homologous chromosomal regions contributing to the development of insulin-dependent diabetes in humans. Mouse models are also stimulating the search for mental illness genes. For example, mouse models have implicated several chromosomal regions in the regulation of alcohol tolerance. The search for homologous regions in humans is ongoing.

Because it is difficult to exactly reproduce a human disease in animals, the results of animal studies must be interpreted with caution. Much of current behavioral genetics research involving mouse models relies on readily observable traits, such as the degree of alcohol tolerance or aggression. These traits are extremely complicated in humans and undoubtedly are under the influence of both genetic and environmental factors. Therefore, translation of research from mice to humans is not straightforward. For example, researchers have bred transgenic and knockout animals that develop amyloid plaques in their brains (the classical hallmarks of Alzheimer disease). However, not all of these animals develop memory impairments later in life. Much work is ongoing to perfect this model. But, despite these cautions about animal models, we anticipate that they will continue to complement work in human genetics.

Disease Genes and Environmental Mechanisms

If you have understood most of what we have written so far in this chapter, it should be clear that molecular genetics studies can find genes and describe the biological mechanisms leading from a genetic mutation to a disease state. But you may be wondering what gene discovery can tell us about the role of the environment in the genesis of psychiatric disorders.

For several reasons, we think that the discovery of genes influencing mental illness and behavior will open new windows for viewing the effects of environmental risk factors. As we noted in prior chapters, we know for certain from twin studies that the environment must play a role in the etiology of mental illness. In some cases adverse environments might cause disorders in the absence of mutant genes. In others, the environment might trigger the effects of a mutant gene. Now we will consider how molecular genetic studies can shed light on each of these possible roles for the environment.

The possibility that adverse environments cause disorders in the absence of mutant genes is a very real one. For example, most people with Alzheimer disease have no affected relatives, suggesting that they may have a nongenetic form of the disorder. But even though this is so, the brain pathology of these isolated cases is identical to that seen for inherited cases of the disorder. Thus, it is likely that the genetic and the nongenetic forms show some similarities in the chain of events leading to disease. Therefore, knowledge regarding the mechanisms of action in familial Alzheimer disease might shed light on the more common nonfamilial Alzheimer disease.

To illustrate this possibility, consider the following hypothetical example. Suppose that studies of the presenilin genes discover abnormal proteins that create amyloid plaques in the brains of Alzheimer disease patients. Perhaps an environmental toxicologist reading about this discovery will recognize the abnormal protein as one that is also created by a toxic compound used in a commercial product commonly found in the home. That would motivate an intense scrutiny of that product, which might eventually lead to the discovery of an environmental cause of Alzheimer disease.

Other strategies can also be used to study the possibility that features of the environment might trigger the effects of a mutant gene. For example, several genetic epidemiologic studies of lung cancer observed the CYP2D6 gene, which controls an enzyme system involved in the metabolism of cancer causing substances. People with one variant of CYP2D6 were less likely to develop lung cancer, even if they smoked, compared with those having another variant, even if they did not smoke. Thus, although smoking is clearly a risk factor for lung cancer, its effects are moderated by our genetic constitution.

The smoking example shows that genes can interact with the environment to cause disease. The study of such interactions is the goal of a branch of human genetics known as *ecogenetics.* Dr. Muin Khoury has shown the potential power of ecogenetic models using mathematical simulations. These indicate that, when genes play a role in the onset of a disorder, their effects will substantially dilute the apparent effects of environmental causes. This means that, in the absence of genetic information, studies of environmental risk factors may erroneously conclude that such factors are either not related to disease or have only a small impact on its onset. These results show that the discovery of disease-producing genotypes will allow us to more accurately estimate the effects of environmental causes.

The ecogenetic framework provides a comprehensive assessment of different types of biologically plausible gene–environment interactions. Table 5.3 describes four common patterns. Each of these patterns assumes that both genes and environment play a role in pathogenesis and that the combination of adverse environment and pathogenic gene always leads to increased risk for adverse outcomes. In the following section we briefly describe these patterns along with examples given by Drs. Ruth Ottman and Muin Khoury

Pattern 1 assumes that both the pathogenic genotype and the environmental pathogen are needed for the disorder to occur. The classic example is phenylketonuria (PKU) which requires both the mutant gene that interferes with the metabolism of phenylalanine and the ingestion of that substance. When this type of gene–environment interaction occurs, the effect of the environment is only seen among people with the patho-

TABLE 5.3. Ecogenetic Patterns of Gene–Environment Interaction

Pattern	Effect of genotype in the absence of environmental risks	Effect of environment in the absence of pathogenic genotype
1	None	None
2	None	Increases risk
3	Increases risk	None
4	Increases risk	Increases risk

Note. Data from Khoury, M. J., Beaty, J. H., & Cohen, B. H. (1993). *Fundamentals of genetic epidemiology.* New York: Oxford University Press.

genic gene and the effect of the gene is only seen among people exposed to the environmental risk factor. The PKU gene was relatively easy to find because phenylalanine is common in the average diet. It would have been much more difficult to find if phenylalanine had been rare.

In pattern 2, the pathogenic genotype exacerbates the effects of the environmental risk factor but has no effect in the absence of that factor. In contrast, the environmental agent increases the risk for illness in the absence of the genotype but its effects are more potent when the genotype is present. This type of gene–environment interaction is seen in the effects of sunlight on skin cancer. Anyone exposed to excessive sunlight increases their risk for skin cancer but this increase in risk is much greater for some genetic types.

Pattern 3 is the converse of pattern 2: the genotype increases risk regardless of the environmental risk factor; the environmental agent exacerbates the outcome of the pathogenic genotype but does not affect outcome in the absence of the genotype.

In pattern 4 both genes and environment increment risk in the absence of the other risk factor but the risk is greatest when both causes are present. An example of this pattern is the interaction between a genetic condition, α-antitrypsin deficiency, and cigarette smoking. Both of these increase the risk for emphysema but the risk is greatest for smokers who also have α_1-antitrypsin deficiency.

When gene–environment interactions occur, the ecogenetic paradigm predicts that studies of genes and environment will show statistically significant effects, but will not be able to provide precise predictions of who is at highest risk for adverse outcomes. Ecogenetic theory predicts that our ability to predict adverse outcomes will increase dramatically if we use statistical models that incorporate gene–environment interactions.

This increase in predictability was shown by Dr. Khoury using statistical simulations. One of his examples is as follows. Suppose that we are evaluating a gene and an environmental factor that interact in accordance with pattern 1. Next assume that the environmental cause leads to a 100-fold increase in the risk for an adverse outcome when the susceptibility gene variant is also present. This 100-fold relative risk will be dramatically underestimated if the gene variant is infrequent. For example, if only 1 percent of people have the variant, then the estimated relative risk for the environmental cause would only be 2.0. At a gene frequency of 10 percent, the estimated relative risk would be 11. Thus, not accounting for relevant genetic variation diminishes our ability to accurately estimate the risk imparted by environmental causes. Dr. Khoury showed similar effects for the other patterns of interaction.

We hope that you now understand how the discovery of psychiatric genes will open new windows for viewing the effects the environment. Once such genes are discovered, we can group patients into those with and those without specific mutations. By studying environmental risk factors in these groups, we should be able to identify potent environmental risk factors that have heretofore escaped detection.

6

Clinical Applications
of Psychiatric Genetics

Counsel woven into the fabric of real life is wisdom.

—WALTER BENJAMIN

Talk that does not end in any kind of action is better suppressed altogether.

—THOMAS CARLYLE

As you have learned in prior chapters, scientists have, for many decades, been studying the genetics of psychiatric disorders. Despite this large body of work, the implications of psychiatric genetic data for clinical work have only recently become apparent. This reflects both increased media attention to genetics and growing sophistication of patients and their families. It also reflects the natural progression of any scientific field: a long period of basic research and development usually precedes clinical applications by many years.

This chapter addresses two clinical uses of genetic data. We first discuss genetic counseling, which provides principles to help clinicians communicate genetic risks to patients and their families. Genetic counseling is well developed, having benefited from the many years' experience of genetic counselors for nonpsychiatric disorders. Then we discuss how psychiatric genetics seeks to improve diagnosis and treatment. A psychiatric genetic approach to diagnosis and treatment is not an alternative to current methods; instead, it provides a set of principles to be integrated into standard assessment and therapeutic paradigms.

159

GENETIC COUNSELING FOR PSYCHIATRIC DISORDERS

Thanks to the diligent efforts of the National Institutes of Health and the biotechnology and pharmaceutical industries, some 4,000 diseases are known to be genetic. Today, diagnostic tests are available for more than 450 genetic disorders. This new knowledge portends hope for many patients and their families as the tree of genetic knowledge bears the fruits of diagnostic and therapeutic applications. But new knowledge creates new confusions. As genetic tests become widely available, their use and interpretation by clinicians will require basic knowledge of human genetic principles and the ability to communicate these principles to patients and their family members. Through genetic counseling we educate our patients about these principles, communicate risks for future disease onset, and correct many of the misconceptions that cause undue distress among people seeking counseling (known as "consultands").

Despite the increasing need for psychiatric genetic counseling, these services are not routinely available at genetic counseling clinics, which focus mainly on rare Mendelian conditions such as Huntington disease and cystic fibrosis. In fact, a survey by the National Institute of Mental Health found that less than 13 percent of members from the National Society of Genetic Counselors had received formal training in psychiatric genetics. The majority of those surveyed rated their knowledge base and ability to provide genetic counseling for psychiatric disorders as no better than "fair or poor."

You might think that standard training in genetic counseling should easily generalize to psychiatric disorders, but you would be mistaken. Certainly, the basic principles of human genetics are the same for all disorders. But medical genetic counseling typically focuses on single-gene disorders and medical genetic counselors often have genetic tests available to guide their estimation of future disease risks. In contrast, as we have emphasized throughout this book, we cannot attribute the familial transmission of psychiatric disorders to single genes. Instead, we must appeal to the notion of complex inheritance whereby the combined actions of many genes and environmental forces lead to mental illness.

Stages of Genetic Counseling

Genetic counseling is most effective when it proceeds systematically through a series of stages. Each successive stage provides you and the consultand with information you both will need for the following stage. During this process you will learn about the consultand and the consultand will learn about the disease that led him or her to seek counseling sessions. In addition to imparting information during each stage, you will be providing the consultand with the psychological and emotional tools he or she needs to enter and complete subsequent stages.

As an aid in describing these stages, we will use two concrete but hypothetical examples. These are based on the following two counseling questions:

Question 1: Jim Sanders is a 35-year-old patient whom you are treating for a severe panic disorder that has plagued him since the age of 16, disrupted his social relationships, and impaired his work performance. He has recently married. He and his spouse want to have children but he keeps putting off a final decision. During a psychotherapy session you discover that Jim's ambivalence has been fueled by a vexing question: Will his children be disabled by panic disorder?

Question 2: Kathy Barrett is a single and healthy 22-year-old college student, she has a brother with schizophrenia, and she participates in your family support groups for schizophrenic patients. One day she asks, "I read in the paper that genes cause schizophrenia. Does that mean I will end up like my schizophrenic brother?"

Both Jim and Kathy need genetic counseling, but each for different reasons. Jim is concerned about making a reproductive choice; Kathy wants information about her own risk for schizophrenia. These are the two main questions addressed by genetic counseling, although other variations do exist. For example, Jim might be concerned about the future of children whom have already been born; Kathy might ask about the risk to children she may someday bear.

In most cases of genetic counseling, the consultand's question usually boils down to: "Will some person (whether already born or not) develop a specific psychiatric disorder?" As you know from reading prior chapters, a simple "yes" or "no" answer will not suffice. An empathic clinician knowledgeable about psychiatric genetics needs to explain the inheritance of mental illness and its implications for the consultand. We call this process "genetic counseling." Its goal is to educate consultands, to provide information about the disorder at hand, to aid the consultand in making important life decisions, and to help consultands cope with the genetic information they receive.

Contemporary genetic counseling should be nondirective. Counselors help consultands understand the nature of genetic conditions and the effects that they will have on affected individuals and their families. Counseling proceeds in a manner that emphasizes the consultand's autonomy and decision-making ability. Genetic counseling can lead consultands to make critical decisions, such as to have or not to have children. It is essential that the counselor's own values about such issues do not influence the course of counseling or the decision of the consultand.

> **Key Point:** The nondirective nature of genetic counseling is as much an ethical issue as it is a clinical one. The ethical counselor provides consultands with the information and tools they need to make crucial life decisions. Counselors should neither make these decisions for consultands nor give their opinions about what choices the consultands should make.

Like Jim Sanders and Kathy Barrett, most consultands seek a simple yes or no answer to a complex question. You must provide an answer that is true to the complexity of the problem yet easy for the consultand to understand. To do so, we suggest you follow the stages of genetic counseling summarized in Table 6.1. If you follow these stages, you will ensure the best outcome for your consultands.

At the outset of counseling, you should review the stages given in Table 6.1 and explain why they are necessary. This provides consultands with a "road map" of the process and assures them that you have a solid rationale for where you plan to take them and how they will get there. You must explain before they embark on the genetic counseling

TABLE 6.1. Stages of Genetic Counseling

1. *Diagnosis.* Verify psychiatric diagnoses in affected individuals.

2. *Family history.* Obtain complete and accurate family history.

3. *Risk of recurrence.* In the absence of a clear mode of transmission, refer to established empirical risks for specific disorders.

4. *Evaluation of the consultand.* Assess consultand's emotional and intellectual capacity prior to proceeding with counseling.

5. *The risk/burden ratio.* Assess consultand's understanding and willingness to negotiate various risks and burdens.

6. *Forming a plan of action.* Help consultand to arrive at a decision most consistent with his or her priorities and world-view.

7. *Follow up.* Continue assessment of the consultand's understanding of pertinent information and follow up life events.

Note. Data from Tsuang, M. T. (1978). Genetic counseling for psychiatric patients and their families. *American Journal of Psychiatry, 135,* 1465–1475.

tour that they will be asked to answer a pivotal question during the counseling process: After having learned about the nature of the disorder and the potential impact of genetic counseling on themselves and their families, do they still want to know the genetic information they originally had requested?

You will need to pose this question because the initial stages of counseling will provide information that may change the consultand's opinion about the desirability of knowing these risks. You should alert the consultand to this future decision point before you start counseling so he or she will not think that, after collecting his or her psychiatric family history, you are making the offer because you have bad news to tell him or her.

Stage 1. Confirm the Diagnosis

Counseling under a mistaken diagnosis is far more dangerous than counseling without knowledge of the underlying mode of transmission. Thus, the counselor first needs to verify the diagnosis of the disorder that led to the consultand's question. It makes no sense to counsel Jim about his children's risk for panic disorder unless we are certain that he actually has panic disorder. The same holds true for Kathy and the schizophrenia that she says afflicts her brother.

For some cases, diagnostic confirmation is straightforward. You yourself may have already diagnosed Jim with panic disorder in a manner that adhered to the criteria and principles of DSM-IV. If so, that would be considered diagnostic confirmation. But if Jim's diagnosis was a "clinical formulation" not rooted in specific criteria or if it was a referral diagnosis of unknown validity, further confirmation would be warranted.

As for Kathy, if you yourself did not diagnose her brother, diagnostic confirmation would be essential. To do so, you should take a cross-sectional clinical picture of her brother along with an assessment of his lifetime course of illness. Do not rely on a referral diagnosis unless you are certain that the referring clinician has rigorously adhered to the diagnostic conventions of DSM-IV or its recent predecessors. Alternatively, the latest version of the International Classification of Diseases (ICD) would also be suitable. We will not review the principles of diagnosis here—these should be well known to most practicing clinicians. If you need to brush up on your diagnostic skills, consult a psychiatry textbook in addition to reading DSM-IV.

Be careful not to underestimate the probability of misdiagnosing patients. Researchers have shown that even in the hands of expert diagnosticians, diagnoses are not 100 percent reliable. In other words, in some cases, even expert clinicians will not agree on a patient's diagnosis. When this occurs, one diagnostician has made an error, despite being as well trained as the other.

> **Clinical Tip:** Do not underestimate the importance of accurate diagnosis. As suggested by the computer science aphorism "garbage in, garbage out," incorrect diagnoses during the initial stage of genetic counseling will make subsequent stages of counseling misleading and perhaps harmful.

Low reliability is a symptom of low diagnostic accuracy. We use the word "accuracy" to indicate the degree to which a diagnosis correctly classifies people who are truly ill and those who are not ill. We use the word "illness" to refer to the "true" but unobservable state of the subject; the word "diagnosis" refers to the results of a diagnostic procedure. Following psychometric and statistical convention, we call this unobservable state of the illness a "latent class." Simple examples of latent classes taken from everyday life reflect the human tendency to classify people according to personality attributes (honest vs. dishonest), emotional states (happy vs. sad), or intellectual ability (intelligent vs. unintelligent). We cannot directly observe honesty, happiness, or intelligence, but we can observe behaviors from which we infer these latent (i.e., unobservable) characteristics.

Like honesty and intelligence, psychiatric diagnoses are unobservable constructs. We can record signs and symptoms and make diagnoses, but we cannot verify them with laboratory tests or pathology reports. We have no way of turning a latent diagnostic class into an observable one. We have no way of knowing for sure if our diagnosis is correct.

Being aware of the existence and causes of diagnostic inaccuracy will help you avoid errors in genetic counseling. Perhaps the most common cause of diagnostic error is lack of information. Some patients are poor reporters of their own symptoms due to psychosis, degraded memory, substance use, or disruptive behavior. Young children may not accurately report internal states, and older children and adults will not accurately recall events from childhood.

Another cause of diagnostic error is "diagnostician drift." This occurs when, with the passage of time and experience, diagnosticians gradually change their method of recording symptoms and integrating them into diagnoses. Drift is especially problematic for psychiatric diagnostic criteria, which can be vague and therefore require a good deal of clinical judgment.

Consider this example. The first DSM-IV criterion for major depressive disorder is "depressed mood most of the day, nearly every day, as indicated by either subjective report (e.g., feels sad or empty) or observation made by others (e.g., appears tearful)." To apply this criterion, the diagnostician must make several judgments: Is the dysphoric mood severe enough to be considered depressed? Does it occur "most" of the day? Does it occur "nearly" every day?

Imagine two diagnosticians who, after having learned to diagnose depression in the same training program, were usually able to agree whether a patient met this first criterion for major depressive disorder. Next imagine that one diagnostician goes on to work for five years in a psychiatric inpatient unit while the other establishes a career as an outpatient psychotherapist in private practice. The former will see very severe cases of depression, the latter will see milder cases. If the two were then asked to diagnose depression in a series of patients, their level of agreement would probably be lower than it had been five years earlier. When compared with the diagnoses of the outpatient psychotherapist, diagnoses made by the inpatient clinician would likely require a greater severity of depression as evidenced by more persistence during the day and over the course of several days. Neither clinician would be "correct" because both would have "drifted" from the diagnostic standard set in their training program. Thus, when you use diagnoses in genetic counseling, you should be aware of how these may have drifted from the "gold standard" diagnoses that are taught in training programs and used in research studies.

Diagnoses for genetic counseling must consider the patient's entire lifetime course. You should strive to avoid allowing your diagnostic impression to be overly influenced by the patient's current clinical state. For example, many patients with bipolar disorder come to clinic for major depressive episodes. A cross-sectional "current" diagnosis would conclude that the patient has major depressive disorder, but a careful lifetime diagnosis would reveal the bipolar disorder. Making such distinctions is essential for meaningful genetic counseling.

When diagnosing people for the purpose of genetic counseling, you should be especially aware of the fact that some psychiatric conditions are mimicked by medical disorders. For example, temporal lobe epilepsy can present as schizophrenia, thyroid disease as depression, and lead poisoning as ADHD. Misdiagnosing medical disorders has two serious implications for Jim Sanders: he will receive the wrong treatment and he will get incorrect information about future risks to his children. Because Kathy Barrett is not ill, the misdiagnosis of her brother will not have treatment implications for her. However, by counseling her in her false identity as the sister of a schizophrenic patient, you will be raising concerns that might otherwise have been alleviated.

Stage 2. Obtain the Family History

The second stage of genetic counseling calls for a comprehensive assessment of the consultand's psychiatric family history. It is not sufficient to know that Kathy Barrett has a schizophrenic brother. We need to know more about other cases of schizophrenia or other disorders that have affected members of her family.

We obtain a family history for three reasons. First, it will provide more information about the diagnosis we have attempted to confirm in Stage 1. For example, by collecting detailed information about Kathy's brother, we will be on a more solid footing when considering his diagnosis. The information that Kathy provides about her brother should not override a better source of information, for example, the brother's medical record, but it should be factored into the process of diagnostic judgment. In some cases, information provided by one relative about another could be crucial for making a diagnosis. Suppose your consultand has a brother who committed suicide. You cannot interview the dead brother and, because he was never treated, he left no medical records. In this case, careful interviews of several relatives would be needed to establish a diagnosis.

> **Clinical Tip:** Semistructured interviews such as the Family History Research Diagnostic Criteria interview or the NIMH Genetics Initiative's Family Interview for Genetic Studies provide a useful framework for family history assessments.

Another reason for taking a family history is to learn about other psychiatric diagnoses in other relatives. This information will provide you with a broad overview of the spectrum of genetic risk in the consultand's family. As we have seen in prior chapters, psychiatric disorders frequently co-occur in individuals and in families. Although a consultand will usually seek advice regarding one disorder, he or she should receive counseling that addresses other disorders in the family. For example, although Jim Sanders may be concerned about his children's risk for panic disorder, you may discover that his wife is an alcoholic and that his own family contains many generations of alcoholics. If that were the case, you might end up telling Jim that his children's risk for alcoholism should be more of a concern than their risk for panic disorder.

The third reason for taking a family history is that you need information about relatives to accurately estimate the risk of concern to the consultand. As you might intuit from the information we provided in previous chapters, the probability of Kathy developing schizophrenia depends not only on whether her brother is truly schizophrenic but also on the presence of other cases of schizophrenia in her family.

We suggest that when you take a family history, you create a pedigree diagram. You have already seen examples of these graphic representations of the family in Figures 4.1a and 4.2a in Chapter 4. A pedigree diagram provides a convenient format for recording diagnostic data that helps you and the consultand visualize the family structure.

Figure 6.1 shows the standard symbols used in pedigree construction. The most frequently used symbols designate diagnosis, gender, and age. For genetic counseling, the pedigree should include all parents, siblings, aunts, uncles, grandparents, and cousins.

Figure 6.2 shows the standard representations for various relationships. For example, in the first panel of the figure, line 1, the relationship line, connects married partners; line 2, the line of descent, connects parents to offspring; and line 3, the sibship line, connects siblings. Line 4 is an individual line designating a member of a sibship.

Figure 6.2 also shows the standard symbols for divorce, consanguinity (e.g., cousin marriages), twin births, no offspring, and adoption. As you can imagine, the correct use of pedigree symbols provides a tremendous amount of information in a small amount of space.

> **Clinical Tip:** To maximize the validity of family history information, use informants who have had substantial contact with the subject; use multiple informants; remember that a diagnosis is more likely to be accurate if the *subject* is currently ill but less accurate if the *informant* is ill; and use less stringent diagnostic criteria than you would when diagnosing someone from a personal interview.

When you construct pedigrees, you must guarantee the confidentiality of the information you gather. What one relative tells you should not be shared with other relations. Assuring confidentiality will increase the likelihood that relatives will provide you with sensitive information such as nonpaternity (e.g., a woman may tell you that her husband is not the father of a child he believes to be his own). The family members you interview will probably not be familiar with diagnostic jargon. Therefore use simple terms to describe the conditions of interest. Structured diagnostic instruments for establishing psychiatric diagnoses in relatives, such as the Family Interview for Genetic Studies (available from the National Institute of Mental Health), are ideal for this purpose.

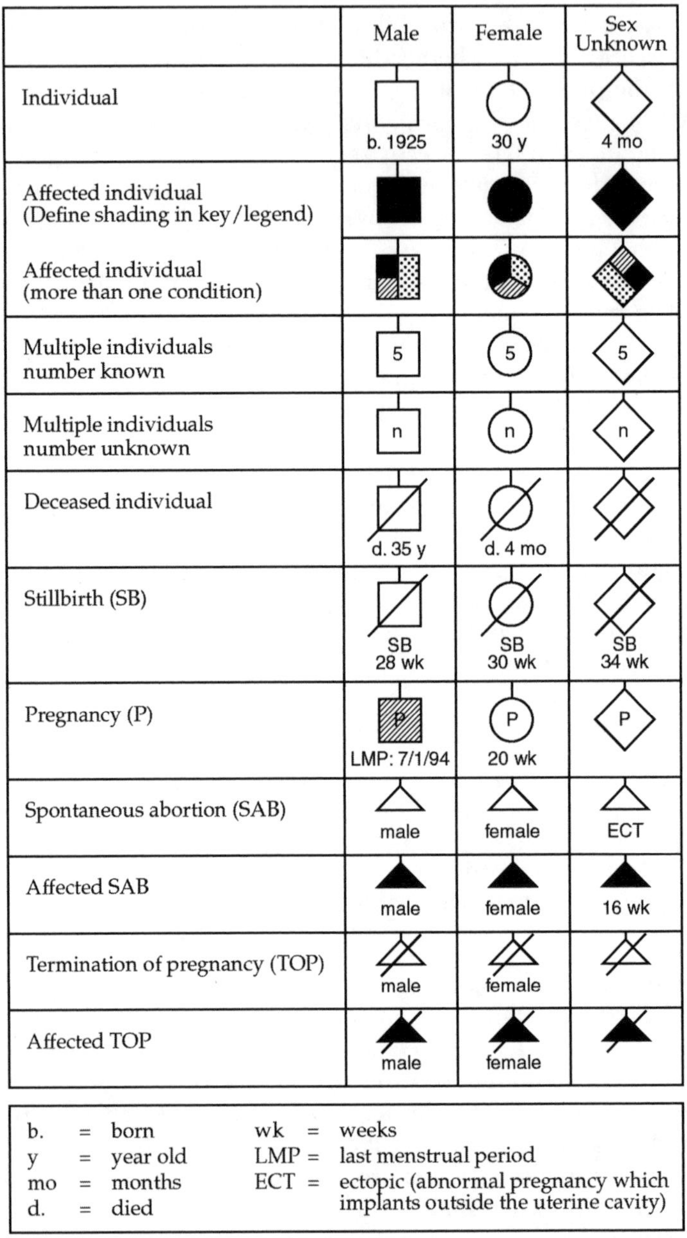

	Male	Female	Sex Unknown
Individual	□ b. 1925	○ 30 y	◇ 4 mo
Affected individual (Define shading in key/legend)	■	●	◆
Affected individual (more than one condition)	▨	◕	◈
Multiple individuals number known	5	5	5
Multiple individuals number unknown	n	n	n
Deceased individual	⊡ d. 35 y	⊘ d. 4 mo	◇
Stillbirth (SB)	⊡ SB 28 wk	⊘ SB 30 wk	◇ SB 34 wk
Pregnancy (P)	P LMP: 7/1/94	P 20 wk	P
Spontaneous abortion (SAB)	△ male	△ female	△ ECT
Affected SAB	▲ male	▲ female	▲ 16 wk
Termination of pregnancy (TOP)	⧄ male	⧄ female	⧄
Affected TOP	◣ male	◣ female	◣

b.	= born	wk	= weeks
y	= year old	LMP	= last menstrual period
mo	= months	ECT	= ectopic (abnormal pregnancy which implants outside the uterine cavity)
d.	= died		

FIGURE 6.1. Common pedigree symbols, definitions, and abbreviations. From Bennett, R. (1995). The genetic family history in primary care. *Genetics Northwest, 10,* 6–10. Copyright 1995 by Robin Bennett. Reprinted by permission.

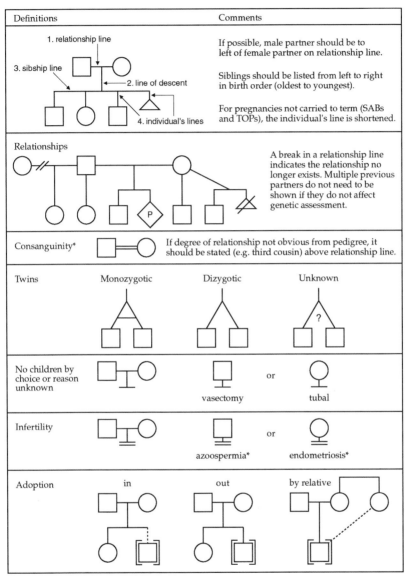

Definitions	Comments

Definitions — 1. relationship line, 3. sibship line, 2. line of descent, 4. individual's lines

If possible, male partner should be to left of female partner on relationship line.

Siblings should be listed from left to right in birth order (oldest to youngest).

For pregnancies not carried to term (SABs and TOPs), the individual's line is shortened.

Relationships

A break in a relationship line indicates the relationship no longer exists. Multiple previous partners do not need to be shown if they do not affect genetic assessment.

Consanguinity*

If degree of relationship not obvious from pedigree, it should be stated (e.g. third cousin) above relationship line.

Twins — Monozygotic, Dizygotic, Unknown

No children by choice or reason unknown — vasectomy, or, tubal

Infertility — azoospermia*, or, endometriosis*

Adoption — in, out, by relative

*Consanguinity - matings between blood relatives.

*Azoospermia - lack of sperms in the semen associated with infertility in men.

*Endometriosis - abnormal growth and function of uterine tissue that may be associated with infertility in women.

FIGURE 6.2. Pedigree line definitions. From Bennett, R. (1995). The genetic family history in primary care. *Genetics Northwest, 10,* 6–10. Copyright 1995 by Robin Bennett. Reprinted by permission.

Stage 3. Assess the Recurrence Risk

Although consultands will often seek an unequivocal yes or no to their counseling question, your answer should be presented in the form of a probability known as the *recurrence risk*, the probability that the disease will recur in a specific family member. You may recall from your mathematics training that a probability is a number between 0 and 1 that expresses the degree of certainty of an outcome. If an event has 0 probability, it will never occur. If its probability is 1, it will definitely occur. If an event is known to occur 50 times for every 100 opportunities, its probability is 0.50 or 50 percent. In genetic counseling, the probabilities of disease usually falls between the two extremes of 0 and 1.

For some psychiatric disorders, the family history may provide information about the mode of inheritance. This can be established by careful examination of the pedigree. For example, some cases of Alzheimer disease are transmitted in an *autosomal dominant manner*, that is, they occur in multiple generations of the same family. Others are either nongenetic or determined by a complex mix of genes and environment. If, while counseling the child of an Alzheimer patient, you found a history of the disease not only in her father but also in her paternal grandmother and that grandmother's father, you would conclude that the disease was autosomal dominant and that her risk for developing Alzheimer disease was high. In contrast, if the consultand's father was the only case in the family, then you would conclude that the father's disease was either nongenetic or complex, and therefore that the consultand's risk was either no greater than the population rate or only slightly elevated.

If you were to find one case of Alzheimer disease in a family, you might be tempted to conclude that the case was not genetic and that the risk to the consultand is zero. For two reasons that conclusion may be wrong. First, even if the case was not at all influenced by genes, the consultand would still be at risk for the same environmental factors that caused the disease in the ill relative. This risk might be very low, but it would not be zero. Second, when a disease has a complex mode of inheritance, many cases do not have affected relatives. Thus, because schizophrenia has a complex mode of inheritance, even if Kathy Barrett's brother was the only schizophrenic in her family, we would not conclude that his disorder was nongenetic. To determine a recurrence risk you will need to rely on either empirical or theoretical risk estimates for specific disorders.

Empirically derived recurrence risks rely on data from family studies of the disorder of interest to the consultand. For example, we know from family studies of schizophrenia that siblings of a patient with schizophrenia have about a 10 percent chance of developing schizophrenia or a related psychotic condition. But before we conclude that this is the correct risk for Kathy Barrett, we would need to consider her age and what is known about the age at onset of schizophrenia. If Kathy is 60 years old, her risk for schizophrenia would be nil because schizophrenia rarely begins so late in life. But if she is 20 years old, her risk is about 10 percent because she is still well within the age range during which onset of schizophrenia can occur. If she is about 30 years old and shows no signs of psychological problems or social dysfunction, her risk would be lower, about 5 percent, because she has survived a good portion of the risk period without any evidence of illness.

The Readings in Psychiatric Genetics section of this book provides many sources that summarize the epidemiologic literature on empirical recurrence risks for psychiatric disorders. These data should be examined before you provide recurrence risk information to consultands.

One problem with empirical recurrence risks is that they are not available for all genetic counseling needs. For example, suppose Kathy Barrett had three cases of schizophrenia in her family: her brother, her father, and a maternal uncle. Because no research study has examined that exact pattern, we cannot provide Kathy with an empirical recurrence risk. Instead, we will need to rely on theoretical recurrence risks.

To compute a precise *theoretical recurrence risk*, we must assume that the disorder has a specific mode of transmission. This poses a problem. Because the mode of inheritance for most psychiatric disorders eludes us, we must approximate the true risk by making assumptions about how these disorders are inherited. Because there is a growing consensus among psychiatric geneticists that few psychiatric disorders are caused by single genes, we should compute risks from the multifactorial model described in prior chapters. Given what we know about the genetics of psychiatric disorders, this model provides a reasonable approximation when exact recurrence risks are not available.

The risk estimates computed from the multifactorial polygenic model are given in Table 6.2. They are calculated from estimates of (1) the disease prevalence in the population and (2) the heritability of the disorder reported from twin studies. The figures in Table 6.2 should be used as guidelines in genetic counseling and should not replace individualized recurrence risk estimates in specific families exhibiting a clear mode of inheritance. They should also not replace empirical recurrence risks when the latter are available.

TABLE 6.2. Theoretical Recurrence Risks for Multifactorial Polygenic Mental Disorders

Disorder	Population rate	Affected parents = 0						Affected parents = 1									Affected parents = 2					
		Affected siblings = 0		1		2		0			1			2			0		1		2	
		U	A	U	A	U	A	U	A ss[b]	A os[b]	U	A ss[b]	A os[b]	U	A ss[b]	A os[b]	U	A	U	A	U	A
Schizophrenia	1%	1	2	6	9	14	18	6	8	15	16	18	25	27	31	36	33	37	42	47	52	57
Bipolar disorder	0.8%	1	2	5	8	13	17	7	6	14	15	17	24	26	29	35	32	36	41	46	51	56
Severe depression Male	4%	3	4	6	8	10	12	7	6	8	10	12	13	15	18	19	13	15	18	21	24	28
Severe depression Female	8%	6	8	11	14	18	21	12	14	15	18	21	22	26	29	30	22	25	33	37	38	41
Alcoholism Male	14%	10	16	22	29	35	42	24	30	32	38	43	45	50	56	57	45	52	57	63	67	72
Alcoholism Female	3%	2	3	5	7	9	11	5	7	8	9	11	12	14	16	17	12	15	17	20	23	26

Note. Risks are shown for a child born into a fmily with two siblings, two parents, and one female second-degree relative. Risks to schizophrenia or bipolar disorder are the same for a male or female at-risk child; population rates are in males and females. When one parent is affected, it is the mother. From Moldin, S. O. (1997). Psychiatric genetic counseling. In S. B. Guze (Ed.), Washington University adult psychiatry (pp. 365–381). St. Louis: Mosby. Copyright 1997 by Mosby. Reprinted by permission.

[a] U, unaffected; A, affected.

[b] ss, same side as affected parent; os, opposite side as affected parent.

Stage 4. Evaluate the Consultand

Before conveying recurrence risks to consultands, you must complete an assessment of their psychiatric features and other psychologic characteristics that might influence what you tell them and how it will be communicated. If the consultand is, like Kathy Barrett, a healthy person asking about her own risk for an illness, you should first complete a standard diagnostic assessment to determine if the consultand already has a diagnosable condition or shows prodromal symptoms of any disorder.

In most cases, such consultands will be free of the illness under investigation. For example, it is unlikely that Kathy Barrett has schizophrenia. But you might find that Kathy has schizotypal personality disorder or that she has experienced brief psychotic symptoms. In addition to pursuing the treatment implications of such symptoms, you will need to determine how they might influence your estimate of the recurrence risk. Based on Kathy's family history of having one schizophrenic brother, you might decide that her risk for schizophrenia is no greater than 10 percent, but if she already has had some psychotic symptoms, your estimate would be greater. Unfortunately, researchers have not yet collected the type of data needed to make accurate predictions in such cases. Instead, you will need to adjust the recurrence risk with clinical judgment informed by knowledge about the patient's specific symptoms and what is known about the natural history of the disorder.

After determining the psychiatric status of consultands, you should determine their mental status. This part of the assessment seeks to answer the question: Will the consultand understand the information that the counseling session will provide? If not, is it possible to educate the consultand so that a meaningful level of understanding can be achieved? In assessing mental status you must first estimate the consultand's overall level of intelligence. From his or her life history or behavior in the clinic, does it appear that he or she will be able to understand the basic concepts of psychiatric genetics that you will need to convey for the consultand to correctly understand the recurrence risk?

In most cases, formal intelligence testing will not be necessary. For example, suppose that Jim Sanders is a successful executive, Kathy Barrett owns her own business, and both show sophisticated communications skills. They will most likely have the intellectual machinery needed to understand the information you plan to convey. But if communication during initial sessions has been difficult or if you have other reasons to suspect a diminished intellectual capacity, then formal intelligence testing might help you tailor your message to the intellectual capacities of the consultand. For example, such testing might show a consultand to have very low verbal skills but average visual–spatial skills. That result would suggest that you need to incorporate visual aids into your presentation of the recurrence risk.

In addition to assessing general intelligence, you need to determine if the consultand understands the concept of probability. You should not take this for granted unless your consultand is a statistician or an insurance actuary. Misunderstanding probability is common. For example, many people are much more nervous about traveling by airplane than they are about traveling by car. This is so even though the probability of dying in an airplane crash is much lower than that of dying in a car crash. And this is not an isolated example. Many people overreact when faced with other low probability adverse outcomes such as death caused by medical error or unforeseen complications during surgeries.

People misunderstand probabilities for two reasons. First, they confuse the intensity of the outcome (e.g., the conflagration caused by an airplane crash) with its probability. Second, they adjust their personal evaluation of the probability based on how much personal control they have over the potential adverse event. This is seen in the anxiety caused by airplane flight. As an airline passenger, we have no control over the success of the flight. The pilot might be tired, the mechanic may have overlooked a point of failure, or wind shear might be lurking in the flight path. In contrast, as the driver of an automobile we have a good deal of control over our fate. We can be vigilant for drunk drivers, drive within the speed limit, and always keep our car in excellent condition.

To many consultands, the prospect of contracting a genetic disorder seems more like flying in a plane that might crash than like driving a car they can control. Thus, you must be alert to the possibility that your estimate of the recurrence risk might not be understood. In fact, you should be prepared to help most consultands understand the concept of probability. You can easily do this with a set of four pennies. Give the pennies to the consultand and have him or her complete the following exercise.

Let's suppose the consultand is a Jim Sanders. Ask him to complete four sets of coin flips. During each set he will be recording the number of times a specified outcome occurs. Each outcome has a precise probability of occurrence which you will tell him prior to the coin flip. By experiencing a range of probabilities, he will develop a more intuitive sense of probability.

Before starting, you need to know the number of children Jim would plan to have if he had no concerns about his children's risk for a psychiatric disorder. Let's call that number n. Then the four sets of coin flips are as follows. Set 1: Flip one coin n times and record the number of times the flip favors heads. For this set, the number of heads represents the number of ill children he might have if the recurrence risk is 50 percent. Have Jim repeat this set 10 times. Each repetition represents a different family of n children who each have a recurrence risk of 50 percent.

These repetitions will show Jim that, although each outcome has a precise probability of occurrence, observed outcomes will vary somewhat from the precise prediction. For example, assume that Jim would like to have four children. Because the probability of heads is 50 percent, four flips of a coin will result in two heads (two ill children) about half the time. But sometimes four flips will yield one or three heads and less commonly will yield no heads or four heads.

When you are sure the consultand understands the results of set 1, proceed to set 2. Flip two coins n times and record the number of times both coins come up heads. For this set, the outcome "two heads" represents an ill child. It has a probability or recurrence risk of 25 percent. We would have Jim flip two coins four times, once for each child he would like to have. Then, as for set 1, he would repeat the process 10 times. These repetitions simulate the range of outcomes produced by a recurrence risk of 25 percent.

The remaining sets proceed in an analogous fashion. For set 3, flip three coins n times and record the number of times all three coins come up heads. The outcome "three heads" represents an ill child. It has a probability or recurrence risk of 13 percent. For set 4, flip four coins n times and record the number of times all four coins come up heads. The outcome "four heads" represents an ill child. It has a probability or recurrence risk of 6 percent. As you go through these sets, have consultands discuss their perceptions of how recurrence risks lead to illness in these "coin families."

> **Clinical Tip:** Most people do not have a clear understanding of probability. Thus, you should plan to spend time using the coin flipping exercises to teach this concept unless you have solid evidence that your consultand grasps probability theory.

The exercise with coin families should leave most consultands with an accurate concept of probability and what it means to say that a disorder will recur in their family with a specific probability. Those who still do not understand should complete 20 repetitions of each set at home. You can discuss the results with them at the next session. If they continue to fail to understand, you may need to determine if there are any cognitive weaknesses or psychological issues that impede their under-standing of probability and recurrence risks.

As you complete your psychiatric and mental status examinations, you should keep the following questions in the back of your mind: How will the genetic counseling information affect the consultand's emotional state? Might it cause a recurrence of dormant psychiatric symptoms? Could it exacerbate an already precarious clinical condi-tion? Will this information diminish the consultand's self-esteem? Will the consultand share counseling information with family members, and will that lead to family conflict or a change in the dynamics of the fam-ily system in which he or she lives?

Do not assume that because the consultand has sought genetic in-formation that he or she has adequately prepared himself or herself for what he or she will learn from the genetic counseling sessions. When you provide genetic information you run the risk of perturbing delicate psychologic and family systems. For example, Kathy Barrett may have developed her sense of self-esteem by contrasting her successes with those of her brother, whose schizophrenia has prevented him from achieving much in life. Indeed, her view of herself as being well ad-justed and her status among family members may hinge on her not hav-ing schizophrenia. Perhaps, having read a magazine article about the disorder, she has sought counseling to allay her fears that she is at risk. If this scenario is true, then the recurrence risk you plan to tell Kathy might adversely affect her.

Understanding the potential perturbations that can be caused by genetic counseling will help you and the consultand deal with them should they arise. For example, you might plan for a subsequent series of personal or family counseling sessions. Whatever you do, do not un-derestimate the potential impact of genetic counseling information. Reactions can be extreme. Consider the sibling of a schizophrenic pa-tient who said that he would rather commit suicide then live in the schizophrenic world that had tortured his sister for many years. This unusual case underscores the necessity for gauging the effects of ge-netic counseling beforehand.

Stage 5. Present the Recurrence Risk

Let's assume that Kathy Barrett and Jim Sanders are intellectually and emotionally capable and that they understand the potential personal and family consequences of receiving genetic information. Because they have decided to continue with counseling, you are now ready to report the recurrence risk. The procedure for doing so will differ for these two cases: Jim needs to understand the recurrence risk in the context of deciding to have children; Kathy needs to understand its implications for her future.

Benefit, Burden, and Reproductive Choice. Helping Jim Sanders make a reproductive choice goes beyond simply telling him what the probability is that his children will have panic disorder. You must also help Jim weigh the potential benefits of having a child against the potential burdens of having an ill child. To do so, Jim must be aware of both these benefits and these burdens and consider them in the context of the recurrence risk you provide.

The benefits of having children will be unique to each consultand; they will vary with the consultand's culture, values, religion, personality, and so on. Moreover, you must address the potential benefits of having children not only with the consultand, but also with the consultand's spouse. Of course, you cannot dictate what these benefits will be. Instead, you should use nondirective interviewing techniques to elicit these benefits from consultands and their spouses. This process may well uncover difficulties in the marriage that need to be addressed with therapeutic interventions before you can obtain a clear understanding of the couple's view of the benefit of having children.

The burden of disease is less idiosyncratic then the benefit of having a child; it refers to the financial, social, and emotional stresses that the disorder would cause in the child and the family. Examples of *financial burdens* include treatment costs for the affected child as well as the family, loss of income due to the need for one parent to stay at home to provide chronic care, and costs of remedial education or private schooling. These costs will, of course, vary with the disease. The costs of having a child with schizophrenia or autism would be much more than those for a child with social phobia.

Social burdens arise from the stigmatization and discrimination associated with psychiatric disorders. Depending on the nature and severity of the condition, people with psychiatric disorders are often shunned by the general public or are made to feel inferior for their handicap. Some families will be prepared to deal with social rejection, others will find it intolerable. Social burdens can be alleviated through family and patient support groups, so these resources should be discussed with the consultand.

Emotional burden refers to the agony and distress that the disorder causes to ill individuals and their family members. In some cases consultands can use their personal experiences to assess these burdens. Jim Sanders has panic disorder, so he understands the personal discomfort of having the disorder. Kathy Barrett, having a schizophrenic brother, knows about the distress caused by living with a psychotic person. For consultands who cannot rely on personal experiences, you must do your best to describe the signs, symptoms, and course of the disorder. For many disorders you can refer consultands to books written for the lay public that provide comprehensive and accessible descriptions of these features.

Once consultands understand the burdens of the disease and their own views of the benefits of having children, you are ready to present the recurrence risk. But before doing so, you should give consultands the option of stopping. At this point in the counseling process you will have taught consultands about the potential impact of counseling on themselves or their families, and about the benefits and burdens associated with the disorder that concerns them. This information may have changed their perceptions of the disorder and may have prompted them to do much soul searching about their views on children. They will also have learned that in the next step you will present them with a recurrence risk, not with a simple yes or no answer to the question: "Should we have children?" These changes may lead some consultands to decline the genetic information you can provide. As we noted earlier, at the outset of counseling it is essential that you alert consultands that this option is available. Then, when you reach this stage of counseling, they will not assume that you are making the offer based on any information you have collected during the counseling process.

The large majority of consultands will choose to continue with counseling. They will be both eager to learn and apprehensive about learning the recurrence risk. After presenting the risk, you should use a probability exercise to clarify the magnitude of risk. If the recurrence risk for the consultand is similar to those simulated by one of the "coin families" you used earlier, then use that coin family to review the magnitude of risk. Otherwise, you can create another coin family that more accurately demonstrates the magnitude of risk.

Consultands should understand two features of the recurrence risk. The risk is an estimate based on research studies and/or theory. It is an estimate, not a certain quantity. You should also tell consultands how the recurrence risk differs from the risk for the disorder in the population at large. The population risk estimate will show them the degree to which their children are at increased risk. For example, we would tell Kathy Barrett that the population risk for schizophrenic disorders is about 1 percent and that her risk is about 10 percent. Thus, she has a tenfold increased risk for the disorder.

A comparison of the recurrence and population risks can provide a useful perspective. For example, a consultand who has a schizophrenic uncle might be horrified to learn that her children are at genetic risk for schizophrenia. She will be somewhat reassured to know that the risk is fairly low (about 3 percent), but will be even more reassured to know that this risk is not much different than that faced by the average person (about 1 percent).

Now that you have communicated the recurrence risk, you must help the consultand integrate this information with the prior discussions of benefit and burden. This can be a complex process. Some disorders have a high recurrence risk but, because they can be effectively treated, do not significantly affect the patient's quality of life. The high risk for such an illness may be viewed as more tolerable than a much lower risk for a disorder that dramatically reduce one's quality of life. For example, a 5 percent risk for a severely debilitating chronic disorder may be perceived as more of a burden to the consultand than a 50 percent risk for a relatively mild episodic disorder. Because there are many combinations of risk, benefit, and burden, genetic counseling must provide a means of quantifying the tolerability of risk for a disease in the context of its burdens and benefits. In doing so, you must also provide consultands with a framework for making key life decisions.

In Jim's case, this process will result in him and his spouse deciding whether or not to have children. As they weigh the burdens against the benefits, you can help in two ways. First, you can use your clinical skills to facilitate the discussion of these issues and to help Jim and his spouse clarify their thinking. Second, you can guide the process by using the simple visual analogy shown in Figure 6.3.

The figure shows a schematic drawing of child's seesaw. Burden sits at one end of the seesaw, Benefit at the other. The recurrence risk enters the picture as the fulcrum (the triangle on which Burden and Benefit are balanced). As the risk increases from 0 to 100 percent, the fulcrum moves from the Burden side of the balance to the Benefit side. In Figure 6.3a, we assume that the consultand's assessment of burden is equal to that of benefit. Because the risk is 50 percent, the two are equally balanced. This means that one decision is as good as the other. But such a balanced situation is unusual. It would be more likely that benefit and burden would not be equal. If the burdens were viewed as greater, then the seesaw would tip toward the Burden side, suggesting that the consultands decide not to have children. If benefits were viewed as greater, they would make the converse decision.

Figure 6.3b shows the case when the risk is less than 50 percent; because Burden is as heavy as Benefit, the seesaw tilts to the right, indicating that Benefit outweighs Burden. This would suggest that deciding to have children would be a good idea. Now imagine that there were few benefits but the burdens were viewed as very large. This would be like having an adult sitting on the Burden side of the seesaw and a small child sitting on the Benefit side. Despite the location of the ful-

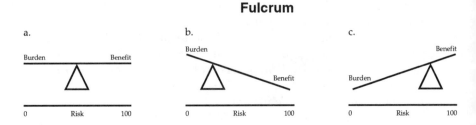

FIGURE 6.3. Weighing risks and benefits in genetic counseling.

crum, the Burden side of the seesaw would go down, suggesting that the consultands decide not to have children.

Figure 6.3c shows what happens when the risk is greater than 50 percent. In this scenario, the benefits would need to be much greater than the burdens for consultands to decide that having children is the best decision.

For psychiatric disorders, recurrence risks to children are less than 50 percent. So consultands will end up pondering the scenario diagrammed in Figure 6.3b. But this will likely change in the future. The discovery of genes that cause psychiatric disorders will allow us to make more refined predictions. When that occurs, it may be possible to predict that some children have a greater than 50 percent risk for becoming ill.

The seesaw analogy in Figure 6.3 provides a useful tool for genetic counseling. Nevertheless, it must be used with caution and clinical sensitivity. As consultands discuss the implications of the model for their decision, you may find them reevaluating their view of benefit and burden. Do not be surprised if consultands disagree with the conclusion reached by the seesaw model. When that happens, it shows that the burdens and benefits have not been adequately assessed.

Suppose that after Jim Sanders gives you his ratings of benefits and burdens, his seesaw model looks like Figure 6.3b, suggesting that he decide to have children. But instead of accepting the logic of the decision (which was based on his own ratings), Jim protests and says it still doesn't feel like the right decision. Thus, there is a conflict between Jim's logical response to the problem and his emotional response. Although his logical ratings of benefit and burden lead to a seesaw model like Figure 6.3b, his emotional responses lead to a model like Figure 6.3c. In this situation, we should work with Jim to help him articulate his emotional responses to the questions of benefit and burden. Then these can be formulated into a seesaw model that he should find acceptable.

Most consultands will understand the difference between their emotional and logical responses to the issues of benefit and burden. When the two disagree, they will be motivated to re-examine their views of this issue. This may lead them to new insights about how they view these issues. For example, maybe Jim has been denying the adverse impact that panic disorder has had on him and his spouse. Although he created a seesaw model using a relatively small estimate of burden, his true view is much larger. This is reflected in his feeling that the model is wrong. Thus, to use the seesaw model successfully, you must use your clinical skills to help consultands work through the psychological issues that prevent them from formulating rational estimates of benefit and burden.

> **Key Point:** As you help consultands make reproductive choices, it is essential that you do so in a nondirective manner. You provide information, not advice; facts not opinions; questions, not answers. You facilitate the consultand's thinking but do not guide it to a conclusion. Throughout this process you must remain alert to the key pitfalls of genetic counselors: as humans, most of us have deeply rooted feelings about the value of children; as mental health professionals, we may have strong opinions about the burdens of psychiatric illness. You must make sure that these values and opinions do not affect your behavior as a genetic counselor.

Counseling Adults at Risk for Psychiatric Disorders. The issues of benefit, burden, and reproductive choice discussed in the prior section do not apply to Kathy Barrett. She is not trying to decide to have children. Instead, she is curious and apprehensive about the possibility that she may someday suffer from the schizophrenia that disables her brother.

For consultands like Kathy, there are no benefits to discuss. But before you present the recurrence risk, you need to be sure that she understands the nature of schizophrenia, its likely course and outcome, and the effectiveness of treatments that are currently available and that might become available in the future. Thus, as you did for Jim Sanders when you discussed the burden side of his decision, you will teach Kathy about schizophrenia and have her talk about her views of the illness. In doing so you will clear up misconceptions and impart knowledge that may allay some of her fears.

Before you teach Kathy about schizophrenia, you should let her discuss her perceptions of the illness and her experience with her brother. This provides you with a view of the disorder through her eyes. Her personal view of schizophrenia will point to areas that you need to emphasize when you teach her the true facts of the disorder. For example, her brother may have a chronic, treatment-resistant form of the disorder that plagues him with chronic hallucinations. She may be relieved to hear that his case is not typical and that even if she has an elevated risk for schizophrenia, her risk for such a pernicious form would be lower.

It is best that this teaching phase of the counseling session precede your presentation of the recurrence risk. Kathy's desire for that information is based upon the knowledge of schizophrenia that she had prior to her genetic counseling. It is possible that, after learning about schizophrenia, she will no longer want to know her degree of risk.

Stage 6. Form a Plan of Action

Genetic counseling does not end with the communication of recurrence risks and the education of consultands about benefit and burden. For many consultands, this process will have implications not only for decisions about childbearing but also for their self-image, social relationships, lifestyle, and plans for the future. Although the first five stages of counseling will prepare both you and the consultand for the potential impact of learning the recurrence risk, new issues may arise. Thus, you must help consultands bridge the gap between the past, when genetic risk was a vague, albeit, palpable concern, and the future, when that risk becomes reified into numerical fact. To do so, you will help them form a plan of action.

For Jim Sanders, the main focus of the plan will be deciding whether or not to have children. Kathy Barrett has no specific decision pending, but the information you have given her may lead her to consider changes in her lifestyle. For example, she may have limited her career options in the belief that schizophrenia would cut short a life of productivity. She may have avoided long-term relationships so as not to burden a spouse in the future. Her risk of about 10 percent may be much lower than she originally perceived. That could lead her to examine career options, consider additional schooling, or lead her to seek a long-term relationship.

Knowledge of genetic risks may affect self-esteem in unknown ways. Jim may feel defective for having "bad genes" and, should he and his spouse decide not to have children, he may feel guilty for denying his wife the joys of raising children. Moreover, Jim and his spouse may go through a period of grief as they deal with the reality that they will not have natural children. Depending upon the nature and severity of such reactions, Jim's plan of action might include psychotherapy or marital counseling sessions. You should also discuss other options with him, such as adoption or impregnation of his wife with donor sperm.

In some cases, the plan of action will include collecting further information about potentially affected relatives. Perhaps, after your best efforts, the only information you could obtain about Kathy's brother is that he is treated with risperidone and was once in a mental hospital for several weeks after the police picked him up for running naked in the streets, screaming at imaginary people. Kathy might decide that she should put more effort into obtaining copies of his medical records, which have been difficult to obtain due to privacy laws in the state where her brother was hospitalized. Thus, her plan would include hiring a lawyer to help her gain access to those records.

Stage 7. Follow Up

After the consultand decides upon a plan of action, you need to provide one or more follow-up sessions to track the implementation of the plan and monitor the consultand for delayed adverse reactions. Typically this involves writing a follow-up letter that summarizes the facts you have conveyed during prior sessions and outlines the plan of action. This letter serves as a written summary for consultands and provides them information to share with interested relatives. The letter also provides a reference for them to consult in the future should they need to refresh their memories about what they learned during the counseling sessions.

A follow-up appointment allows continued assessment of the consultand's understanding of the previous discussions. In addition, it gives the clinician time to obtain more information, such as subsequent births or the onset of disease in other family members. If the mode of inheritance becomes apparent with this additional information, then recurrence risks should be revised for greater accuracy.

A Case Study

In general, four types of individuals seek psychiatric genetic counseling: the patients themselves, the families of patients, the spouses of patients, and prospective adoptive parents. The pedigree in Figure 6.4 will be used to illustrate the genetic counseling of a hypothetical consultand. The numbers below the individual symbols refer to the current age or age at death for each family member.

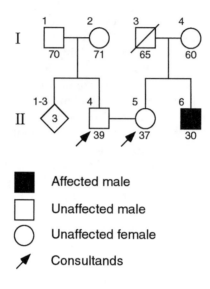

FIGURE 6.4. Hypothetical pedigree.

The pedigree illustrates the case of Mr. and Mrs. M, a couple in their late 30's who are trying to decide if they should have children. Mrs. M's brother (pedigree symbol II-6) was diagnosed as schizophrenic in his teens and has been hospitalized many times for treatment of auditory hallucinations and delusions of persecution. The couple is worried that their future offspring will develop schizophrenia. To the best of their knowledge, there are no other affected family members. However, since Mrs. M's father was adopted, the family history from his side of the family is unknown. For this couple, the seven stages of genetic counseling are as follows.

Stage 1: Diagnostic Confirmation

We first verify the diagnosis of schizophrenia in the affected brother by reviewing all his psychiatric and medical records. Fortunately, he is willing to be interviewed, but the interview leaves us perplexed. Because he is a poor historian, we cannot reconstruct his psychiatric history. Moreover, during the interview he shows signs of mania, which lead us to suspect that the presumed diagnosis of schizophrenia was wrong.

To help us solve this puzzle, we request the medical records from his prior hospitalizations. Because he had been hospitalized at several different hospitals in four different states, the collection of records takes several weeks. Nevertheless, it is worth the effort because the records show that the brother has been ill since age 18 and has been hospitalized 10 times for acute episodes marked by auditory hallucinations and paranoid delusions. None of these episodes show any dysregulation of mood, suggesting that our suspicions of mania were unfounded. In between psychotic episodes, he is stable on risperidone but is unable to work due to severe symptoms of social withdrawal, anhedonia, and poverty of thought. He spends most of his time at home in the care of his elderly parents.

Stage 2: Family History

We interview both the husband and the wife to obtain their own psychiatric histories and additional family history. It is especially important to determine if either of Mrs. M's parents were affected, preferably through personal interviews of her mother, if possible. The husband's psychiatric history reveals a history of heavy alcohol use but no evidence of abuse or dependence in him or other family members. Mrs. M's family psychiatric history reveals possible schizotypal personality disorder in her father and three episodes of mild depression in her mother, who never sought psychiatric treatment.

Stage 3: Risk of Recurrence

Because her brother clearly has schizophrenia and her father is possibly affected with a schizophrenia spectrum disorder, Mrs. M's family appears to have a genetic liability for schizophrenia. Although Mrs. M's mother has a history of mild recurrent depression, the mild nature of her syndrome and the lack of depression in other family members leads us not to be concerned about the potential genetic risk for depression. The father's history of heavy alcohol use is a concern, but given that it too was mild, we decide to focus our counseling efforts on the risk for schizophrenia. We do, however, discuss these other disorders and suggest that the couple be alert to their signs and symptoms in themselves and their relatives. Further evidence of these disorders in the family would be grounds for seeking additional genetic counseling.

When we address the recurrence risk for schizophrenia, we decide to use the theoretical estimates from Table 6.2. With an affected second-degree relative (the brother), the risk for schizophrenia to an offspring of Mr. and Mrs. M is low, about 2 percent. We found this number as follows. From the top of the table, we choose the "0" label under the heading "Affected Parents," because both Mr. and Mrs. M are not affected. This restricts our search to the left side of the table (i.e., the first six columns of recurrence risks). Next, under the heading "Affected Siblings," we choose "0" because the Ms have no affected children. This further restricts our search to the first two columns. Finally, from these two columns we choose the column labeled "A" because a second-degree relative of the potential child is known to be affected.

By perusing Table 6.2, you can see how the recurrence risk changes with the pattern of illness in the family. For example, suppose Mrs. M had a schizophrenic disorder. We would then choose 1 under Affected Parents, 0 under Affected Siblings, and the "ss" column under "A" for second-degree relatives. We choose "ss" because the affected second-degree relative (Mrs. Ms brother) comes from the same side of the family as the affected parent (Mrs. M). Thus, the risk to the child is about 8 percent. As you inspect this table, please remember that it only provides a rough guide. Accurate recurrence risks for genetic counseling should be informed with knowledge about the empirical recurrence risks for the disorder of interest.

Stage 4: Evaluation of the Consultand

Both consultands are college-educated professionals. They have excellent verbal skills and are clearly able to understand the nature of the information to be provided. No further mental status testing is required. These consultands purport to understand the concept of probability, but we nevertheless proceed with the coin flip exercise. Mr. M finds this to be a very useful process and is pleased to repeat the process at home. By the end of this stage, they have acquired the concept of probability needed for counseling.

Due to the demands of their careers, childrearing has been postponed. Intellectually, they understand the necessity for the delay, but Mrs. M is concerned that she is passing the "prime years of childbearing." Mrs. M also has had significant difficulty coping with her brother's illness, his lack of employability, and his continual dependence on their mother. She admits that she would have considerable difficulty dealing with an affected child.

Mr. M dearly desires children. Having been raised in a traditional family, he has been frustrated by his wife's unwillingness to compromise her career for the sake of having children. He views her need for genetic counseling as simply one more delaying tactic. The couple's discussion of this issue shows it to be a source of persistent acrimony in their relationship. Moreover, Mr. M's opinions have gradually eroded Mrs. M's self-esteem, a process that has been exacerbated by Mrs. M's belief that she is genetically defective. Thus, she finds herself in a quandary: to not have children, which could destroy her marriage, or to bear children who may suffer a devastating disease.

In this case, evaluating the consultands reveals that counseling has the potential for perturbing the marital relationship. It may change Mrs. M's view of herself for better or worse, making it essential that she and her husband have a clear understanding of the information to be presented. Mr. M's response to counseling will likely be influenced by his unsophisticated understanding of his wife's dilemma. Follow-up sessions, and perhaps marital therapy, will be needed to assure that counseling does not destabilize their marriage.

Stage 5: Presentation of the Recurrence Risk

The consultands easily discuss their views of why children are desirable. Both have cultural backgrounds that view parenting as an important part of marriage and both have experienced the joys of being around children through visits to friends and relatives. They know less about the burdens of schizophrenia, so we spend a considerable amount of time describing the disorder. We have them read the book *Schizophrenia: The Facts* and spend an entire session discussing its contents and answering questions. Mr. M searches for information on the Internet and deluges us with many sophisticated questions about the disorder's causes and potential outcomes. When the discussion of benefits and burdens has been completed, we remind the couple that we have reached a decision point: Do they want to continue with genetic counseling? Do they want to learn the recurrence risk? They do.

Mr. and Mrs. M are both surprised that their offspring's risk for schizophrenia is so low. They had expected that each child would have a "fifty–fifty" chance, so they are very much relieved. Finding the see-saw analogy very useful, they quickly decide that benefit outweighs burden, a fact that clearly delights Mr. M and seems to have brought the couple closer to one another. We encourage their positive attitudes but also suggest that they spend a week thinking about their decision so that they can form a more detailed plan of action.

Stage 6: Formation of a Plan of Action

By their next session, the Ms have further strengthened their resolve to have a child. They have been working out a timetable and spend much of the session revising details. Despite their optimism, they recognize the need for further counseling and arrange for follow-up sessions of marital therapy.

Stage 7: Follow Up

The follow-up letter is sent to the consultands within one week. In plain language, the letter recaps the content of the counseling sessions, and presents both the recurrence risk and population prevalence of schizophrenia. The letter describes the plan of action and ends by noting that further genetic counseling is available should the need arise.

IMPLICATIONS FOR DIAGNOSIS AND TREATMENT

In addition to making genetic counseling possible, psychiatric genetic data have implications for the diagnosis and treatment of the mentally ill. In the future, as genes are discovered and their mechanisms of action better understood, psychiatric genetics will have a tremendous impact on clinical practice. DNA tests will be available to aid genetic counselors and to diagnoses disease. The delineation of subforms having different genetic and environmental contributions will allow clinicians to target treatments to specific causes. And, perhaps, the technology of gene therapy will allow physicians to prevent psychiatric disorders at the very earliest stages of life. We discuss these potential future developments in the subsequent chapter. Here we show how current psychiatric genetic knowledge can facilitate diagnosis and treatment.

> **Key Point:** The implications of psychiatric genetics for diagnosis and treatment are only now emerging from the research literature. Much more work is needed to create consensus guidelines for clinical care. Until then, the principles discussed in this section, along with knowledge of the psychiatric genetic literature, will provide a framework for incorporating psychiatric genetic knowledge into clinical care.

Family-Based Diagnosis

Any working clinician knows that psychiatric diagnoses are not always clear: patients may be poor reporters, records from prior mental health contacts may not be available, or the patient may be in the early phases of a disorder that cannot be identified. In these situations, the fact that most psychiatric disorders are familial raises the clinical question: Could diagnoses in relatives clarify ambiguous diagnoses in our patients?

Well, if we believe that the diagnoses of relatives are useful in pre-dicting the risk for illness in children yet to be born, it naturally follows that they should provide some information about the ambiguous diag-noses of living family members. Thus, in some cases, by determining what psychiatric illnesses occur in the patient's family, clinicians may be more precise in the diagnosis of the patient.

> **Key Point:** In some families, a clear diagnosis in one family member may provide clues to the nature of an ambiguous disorder affecting a relative having an atypical clinical presentation.

For this purpose, the psychiatric family history is most useful for "atypical" cases or when little data about the patient is available. The use of family history data is straightforward and intuitive. For example, consider the case of a 30-year-old patient admitted to a hospital who has no prior psychiatric history. He shows both the psychotic symp-toms of schizophrenia and the affective symptoms of bipolar disorder, without clearly meeting criteria for any disorder. If the patient has two siblings with bipolar disorder, the diagnosis of bipolar disorder would certainly be suspected. If these siblings were schizophrenic, the diagno-sis of schizophrenia would merit more attention.

But one must be cautious in using family history to formulate diag-noses. One technical point is that the DSM-IV diagnostic nomenclature has no provisions for incorporating family history into the diagnostic process. Moreover, because there is little research on this topic, we do not know the ultimate value of family-based diagnoses. Thus, taking a family history may increase or decrease your suspicions about specific diagnoses, but it cannot be used as a diagnostic criterion.

Moreover, it is certainly possible that a person with two schizo-phrenic siblings happens to have bipolar disorder. So the latter diagno-sis should not be ruled out, especially if the predominance of data about the patient support its validity. Thus, any family-based diagnosis must be considered provisional. Such a diagnosis provides clinical hy-potheses to be tested by collecting more comprehensive information about the patient to be diagnosed.

Of course, family-based diagnosis cannot replace the careful docu-mentation of psychopathology and its course that will eventually clarify ambiguous diagnoses. But when diagnostic data are lean and clinical decisions must be made, knowledge of psychiatric genetics can lead to more accurate provisional diagnoses. In some cases, the benefit to the patient could be substantial. The differential diagnosis of schizophrenia and bipolar disorder is paradigmatic. For both disorders, research suggests that early pharmacologic treatment can mitigate the course of illness. The basic idea is that untreated episodes of illness harm the brain in a manner that makes it more susceptible to subsequent episodes and a chronic course of illness and disability. Thus, the correct treatment at the first onset of symptoms may reduce the patient's degree of lifelong suffering. Because family-based diagnosis can clarify ambiguous diagnoses, it can help patients by improving the accuracy of early treatment decisions.

As we discussed in prior chapters, our diagnoses of patients must be alert to the potential for *psychiatric comorbidity,* the tendency for patients with one psychiatric disorder to also have another. In this context, the ubiquity of comorbidity should lead us to suspect that patients we have diagnosed with one disorder may harbor the familial vulnerability to another, even though that other disorder is not clinically evident.

For example, suppose you receive a new referral, Boris Strelnikov, who without question meets diagnostic criteria for alcohol abuse. It is very unlikely that information about his relatives would lead you to change his diagnosis, but that data might nevertheless be useful. For example, suppose you find that Boris has a mother who is being treated for panic disorder and a brother who suffers from limited symptom panic attacks. This should make you suspect that Boris harbors the familial predisposition to panic disorder. Moreover, it should encourage you to delve more deeply into his personal history of panic symptoms. This inquiry could lead you to discover that he had had some of these symptoms in the past, but these symptoms have since been obscured by alcohol use. If this makes you suspect that Boris uses alcohol to control panic symptoms, it will likely influence your treatment planning.

In addition to clarifying the diagnoses and vulnerabilities of your patients, diagnoses of family members will teach you a good deal about the family your patient must deal with. For example, suppose you are treating Dolores Rialto for major depression. Now consider two alternative scenarios: (1) she has three healthy young children and a husband who shows no signs of psychiatric impairment and (2) she has two healthy children, one son with ADHD, and a husband with antisocial personality disorder. It is self-evident that treatment planning for Dolores must consider the diagnoses of family members. They might suggest the need for family treatment or for the individual treatment of family members.

In some cases, you will find that the treatment of "discovered" disorders in family members has more of an impact on your initial patient than their own treatment. For example, perhaps Dolores was refractory to both medications and cognitive therapy but the discovery of ADHD in her son led to him receiving an effective course of stimulant treatment. The subsequent reduction of chaos in the home could help Dolores by removing a source of chronic stress and demoralization.

Fighting Therapeutic Nihilism

During the past three decades, the scientific revolution of biologic psychiatry has yielded many advances in the treatment of mental illness. For a wide range of conditions—including chronic disabling disorders such as schizophrenia and milder, episodic ones such as panic disorder—biologic treatments have shown a remarkable degree of efficacy. Although these advances cannot be denied, they have left some patients with what Paul Meehl called "therapeutic nihilism"—the belief that only biologic treatments can help persons afflicted with "genetic" or "biologic" disorders.

Therapeutic nihilism inhibits the full recovery of patients. Many patients suffer severe blows to their self-esteem upon learning that they are "biologically defective." The wounds inflicted by these blows heal slowly in a competitive public prone to categorize people as normal or abnormal, successes or failures, good or bad. It is, perhaps, unfortunate, that discussions of mental illness so frequently use the dichotomy of normal versus abnormal, that college courses about psychopathology are often named "Abnormal Psychology," and that the word "abnormal" is used in the titles of scientific journals about mental illness.

Of course, mental illness had been stigmatized centuries before biologic psychiatry was born. But under the new regime of biologic psychiatry, the stigma of mental illness takes on a new guise and affects patients in different ways. For some patients, the very idea that they are "abnormal" can be demoralizing. But to view this as a genetic defect renders it an immutable fact of their biologic essence. Medicines might mitigate symptoms, but they will not fix aberrant genes.

Some patients think this way because they have a primitive, media-driven knowledge of mental illness. Thus, the best way to combat cases of self-stigmatization is to educate the patient about his or her disorder and the complexity of its etiology. This process should help the patient understand key facts about his or her mental illness: (1) its multifactorial nature, (2) the role of the environment, (3) the role of the self, and (4) dimensions of liability.

By educating the patient within the framework of the multifactorial model, you will prepare him or her for understanding what we mean by "dimensions of liability." This concept derives from the multifactorial model's assumption that each of us has an unobservable "liability," or predisposition, to develop mental illnesses. As you may recall from prior chapters, this liability, like height, varies from low to high, with many intermediate values. Thus, much as there is no absolute definition of who is tall and who is small, the multifactorial framework does not classify people as "normal" or "abnormal."

Your goal in presenting the multifactorial model to patients is simple: you want them to understand that their problems are not caused by a simple biologic switch that was turned on at birth. You want them to view their current problems as one of many designs woven into the larger tapestry of their human experience. Flaws in this tapestry can be repaired with the threads of biology, psychological development, insight, spiritual expression, and critical life events.

Your discussion of the multifactorial theory of disease sets the stage for helping patients understand the role of the many factors that lead to disease and foster recovery. Ideally, it would be best to use examples that are specific to the disorder that afflicts the patient. But when that is not possible, showing them the results of twin studies should clarify this point. When patients realize that genetically identical twins are not always both affected with their disorder, they can better appreciate the impact that the environment may have had on their own problems.

At this point in the patient's education, you will have begun to shift his or her attributions about the cause of his or her illness from a simple genetic defect to a broader source of genes and adverse environmental events. The next step is to explore the role that the self plays in the patient's structure of attributions. Patients who hold primitive theories of biological causation can develop what Dr. Martin Seligman called "learned helplessness," the belief that they cannot control the course of events in their lives. Such reasoning is not sound. It assumes that having a biologic defect means that a patient's personality, temperament, cognition, and behavior cannot influence the course of his or her disorder.

Learned helplessness can have profound implications. Not only can it lead to demoralization and clinical depression, but it can also make patients not consider alternative or adjunctive treatments. This is ultimately counterproductive: a young schizophrenic patient will not attend social skills training sessions, an attorney with panic disorder will opt out of behavior therapy, and a periodically depressed mother will decline cognitive therapy. These patients believe that psychosocial treatments cannot help them because they have a biologic disease.

Such patients need to understand that the self and its expression is a very powerful source of environmental influence. The schizophrenic patient can learn to modulate his exposure to overstimulating environments that worsen this psychosis. The attorney with panic disorder can unlearn phobias that have impaired her practice. The depressed mom can restructure the way she thinks about her world to protect her from future depressions.

Perhaps the easiest way to teach patients the role of the self is to use examples of medical disorders. Like psychiatric disorders, many cases of coronary heart disease are multifactorial. A combination of predisposing genes, a high-fat diet, and lack of exercise leads to hypercholesterolimia and heart attacks. Yes, these patients have a biological defect and yes, they can be treated with lipid-lowering drugs. But such patients can also reduce the amount of cholesterol in their diets and increase their amount of exercise. These activities of the "self" can reduce their cholesterol levels and prevent heart attacks.

Facilitating Treatment

In addition to helping patients overcome therapeutic nihilism, there are other ways in which psychiatric genetic knowledge can facilitate the treatment of mental illness. One possibility derives from a subdiscipline known as pharmacogenetics, which studies how genetic variation affects how people metabolize and respond to medicine. Here we are not concerned with the use of pharmacogenetics for understanding metabolic differences. These findings are well documented and available to practicing psychopharmacologists.

Instead, we will focus on the potential for pharmacogenetic data to guide the choice of drugs. Ideally, we would be able to show which specific genetic variants predict good and poor responses to specific agents for specific disorders. For example, some studies suggest that abnormalities in genes for serotonin receptors may predict which schizophrenic patients show a good response to the atypical antipsychotic drug clozapine. This is, however, an emerging field with very limited data. Thus, we cannot make any specific recommendations.

There are, however, data suggesting that, if a patient has relatives with the same disorder, the relative's response to specific biologic treatments should be considered in choosing a therapy for the patient. The relevant data are not extensive, but there have been several studies of mood disorders that have implications for clinical practice.

There is some evidence that bipolar patients with a family history of bipolar disorder are more responsive to lithium than those without a family history of the illness. There are also studies of depression suggesting that antidepressant response runs in families. That is, if an antidepressant is effective for one depressed patient, it is likely to be effective for a biologic relative. But, since little is know about the familial transmission of treatment response, the use of family data in treatment should be flexible and should not override other considerations that have been more extensively researched.

Another use for genetic findings is in the area of medication compliance. Many patients are reluctant to take psychotropic medication and others find it difficult to maintain their prescribed regimen. These problems are mitigated by discussing the genetic etiology of a disorder when teaching a patient about his or her illness. Many patients hold naïve beliefs about the etiology of their disorder; they are quick to attribute it to life circumstances, events in the past, or their own psychologic inadequacies. Although such factors should not be summarily dismissed, they may make it difficult for patients to accept the biologic component to their problems.

For many psychiatric disorders genetic data, described in the context of the multifactorial model of inheritance, provide the quickest and most convincing means of showing patients how biology plays a role in their condition. Although this is often easier when other relatives are known to be ill, it is also useful when the patient is the only family member affected.

You can also use genetic data as part of the educational component to family therapy, especially for those therapies that do not assume that the illness was directly or indirectly *caused* by deviant family interaction. This educational use of psychiatric genetic knowledge attempts to reduce the family's self-blame for the illness. Once families learn about the genetic and biologic bases of the illness, they can discard guilty feelings and more productively cooperate in the treatment of their relative. Understanding biologic bases also helps families accept the necessity of medication.

Family therapists will also find it useful to complete a comprehensive assessment of family members for mental illness and spectrum conditions. Given that most mental illnesses run in families, it makes little sense to view the initially referred family member as the "patient" and other members as contributing to the patient's illness or recovery through their interactions. In fact, you will likely find that most families have more than one ill member as well as others who may have spectrum conditions.

For example, Tony Gianelli is a 6-year-old boy who clearly has ADHD. His family has been referred for family therapy. Although there are many approaches to the family therapy of ADHD, typical strategies would be to teach behavior management skills to the parents; to teach cognitive skills to Tony to help him gain better control of his impulsivity, inattention, and hyperactivity; and to work with the family to change maladaptive patterns that might be facilitating Tony's problems.

Now, imagine two scenarios. In the first, a genetically uninformed therapist proceeds with therapy following the usual guidelines for his or her therapeutic approach. In the second, a genetically informed therapist—alert to ADHD's known familial transmission and co-transmission with other disorders—completes a family psychiatric history. The first therapist works without knowledge of other disorders in the family. The second learns that the father also has ADHD and abuses alcohol. Moreover, the mother has had recurrent episodes of depression.

The latter therapist will likely be more effective than the former. The family psychiatric history would likely be valuable for several reasons. It may be necessary to deal with the parental disorders before attempting any family therapy. An active alcoholic disabled by symptoms of ADHD is not a good candidate for learning behavior management skills. In some cases, treating parental disorders may be a prerequisite for successful family therapy

Of course, the genetically uninformed therapist may learn of these other disorders. But that could create other problems. Some genetically uninformed family therapy systems will attribute one family member's psychopathology to the environmental effects of being exposed to another's psychopathology rather than to the shared genes that put family members at risk for both disorders. Here is one illustration. Some therapists may attribute maternal depression to the effects of raising an ADHD child. If so, their family therapy goal may be to teach the mom better coping skills and to recommend medication for the child. The implicit assumption is that the child's disorder is biologic and is driving the mother's condition. But the reverse my be true or, more likely, both family members are suffering from a genetically mediated condition that is exacerbated by environmental events.

The implications of genetic data for diagnosis and treatment are speculative. Notably, there is almost no research directly addressing these issues. Thus, we must rely on clinical experience as well as inferences from what we have learned from psychiatric genetic research. Like most fields, clinical applications emerge during the mature phases of a scientific discipline. Because psychiatric genetics is entering that phase, you can expect more clinical applications to be tested in the future. Indeed, the future of psychiatric genetics will answer many scientific and clinical questions. It will also raise many questions about the legal, ethical, and social implications of those answers. So, having reviewed the past and its implications for the present, our final chapter looks into the future of our discipline and its potential for further improving the care of our patients.

7

The Future
of Psychiatric Genetics

*It is possible to believe that all the past is but the beginning of a
beginning, and that all that is and has been is but the twilight of
the dawn. It is possible to believe that all the human mind has
ever accomplished is but the dream before the awakening.*

—H. G. WELLS

*B*y now, you have learned much about the theories, methods,
findings, and clinical implications of psychiatric genetics. Of course,
given that there has been a century of research on the topic, we have
only been able to emphasize the basics, the tip of the proverbial ice-
berg. Nevertheless, these fundamentals provide a solid foundation of
knowledge concerning what you and your patients will face in the future.

What the future will bring we cannot predict with certainty. Undoubtedly, a contemporary H. G. Wells could imagine a world transformed by snippets of DNA yet to be discovered: genes that cause
mental illness, mold personality, foster intelligence, strengthen the
super ego, create criminals. . . . Could there be a world in which a
supercomputer assays our genetic profile at birth and tattoos it on our
back? Would that profile help physicians heal babies before they become ill? Would it be used to discriminate against those deemed genetically inferior by some Orwellian bureaucracy?

Although this science fiction could become science fact, rampant

196

speculation exceeds the scope of this chapter. Instead, we will explore three potential challenges that psychiatric genetics faces now as it heads into the future: the creation of new technologies for gene finding, the diagnostic and therapeutic use of the mental illness genes that will someday be discovered, and the ethical, legal, and social implications of knowing who is and who is not at genetic risk for psychopathology.

THE PROMISE OF NEW TECHNOLOGIES

Molecular Genetics: The Human Genome Project

Following the advice of many scientists, in 1988 the U.S. government sent the following directive to the Department of Energy and the National Institutes of Health: by the year 2005, describe the entire sequence of DNA that constitutes the human genome. Dubbed the Human Genome Project, and complemented by parallel projects in Asia and Europe, this multibillion dollar international scientific effort may eclipse the Moon landing as the greatest scientific achievement of this century.

Consider this: The human genome comprises 3,000,000,000 base-pairs. About 2,850,000,000 base-pairs are "junk" DNA, the detritus of evolution, useful for creating genetic markers but holding no clues to the structure and function of the human body in either health or illness. Hidden within this junk pile are about 150,000,000 base-pairs that are the building blocks of some 100,000 genes. The Human Genome Project seeks to separate the genes from the junk while describing each in exquisite chemical detail. Though a formidable task, project officials have announced that it should be completed in 2003, two years ahead of schedule.

Key Point: The completion of the Human Genome Project will be the geneticists' equivalent of landing a person on the Moon. Through the concerted efforts of hundreds of scientists, this federally funded project will provide a complete description of the human chromosomes.

As you know from the chapter on molecular genetics, scientists find genes through linkage analysis by using a map of genetic markers. Many of these markers were by-products of the Human Genome Project and even more are in development. Remember, the power of a linkage study increases with the variability of markers (i.e., how many different versions there are) and the proximity of markers to the unknown gene. Thus, the more milestones we have on the genomic highway, the easier our task will be to find genes along the way. Every two years, the Human Genome Project supports Human Genome Mapping workshops. These provide scientists with a forum in which to catalogue genetic milestones in a manner that makes the genetic map more accessible to their peers.

But the vision of the Human Genome Project extends far beyond the creation of bigger and better maps. As project scientists sequence the base-pairs that constitute our genome, they will discover a wealth of information about the structure of genes and their function in the human body. These scientists are also mapping and sequencing the genomes of other organisms, most notably mice and bacteria. Soon the ability to make comparisons between species may yield insights into how genes function in humans.

As you can imagine, this attempt to sequence three billion base-pairs and create thousands of markers requires advanced computer systems, data storage and retrieval methods, and statistical procedures. Thus, the Human Genome Project has set aside funds not only for laboratory studies of genes, but also for developing the computational and statistical procedures that are needed to store, analyze, and disseminate the mountain of data generated by the project.

Because many scientists will be needed to complete the project and to follow up on its many discoveries, the Human Genome Project was also given a mandate to support the training of junior scientists at both the pre- and postdoctoral levels. Creating a new and larger cadre of molecular genetic and biomedical scientists will help the project achieve another goal: to develop innovative technologies that have practical implications for both the practice of medicine and the use of genetic technology in industry. In this respect, the Human Genome Project is very much like NASA's space exploration programs. The technologies NASA created to send people to the Moon and probes to Mars have had many uses on Earth. We can expect similar contributions from the technological innovations of the Human Genome Project.

From the perspective of psychiatric genetics, the Human Genome Project is an immense factory producing and refining the tools we will need to discover the genes that cause mental illness. These tools come in the form of improved genetic markers, faster methods of genotyping, denser genetic maps, and better statistical methods for the analysis of complex genetic diseases. Will these new high-tech tools be sufficient for finding mental illness genes? Or do we also need to improve the low-tech tools of psychiatric diagnosis and clinical nosology?

A Clinical Nosology for Psychiatric Genetics

In the chapter about molecular genetics, we implicitly assumed that clinical methods used to classify family members as ill or well were correct. At face value, this assumption seems reasonable. After all, many years of clinical observation and systematic research were used to create the American Psychiatric Association's *Diagnostic and Statistical Manual of Mental Disorders* (DSM) and the World Health Organization's *International Classification of Diseases* (ICD). These diagnoses are used around the world to guide clinical practice and systematize psychiatric research. Moreover, since many of these diagnoses are known to be heritable, shouldn't they be useful for genetic studies?

The answer to this question boils down to one word: heterogeneity. Recall the two dimensions of heterogeneity from Chapter 3: causal and clinical. *Causal heterogeneity* occurs when two or more causes can, on their own, lead to the same clinical syndrome; *clinical heterogeneity* occurs when a single cause leads to more than one clinical condition. We described these dimensions of heterogeneity in Figure 3.1 (refer back to p. 47 in Chapter 3).

In the figure, the "Full Disorder" (the smaller, shaded circle) represents the disorder as diagnosed by one of the official diagnostic systems. But as the figure suggests, this condition only partially overlaps with the larger circle, which represents the full spectrum of conditions caused by the disease genes. Ideally, psychiatric geneticists could select families for genetic studies using a nosology that corresponded to the larger, not the smaller, circle.

We call such a nosology a "psychiatric genetic nosology." It would be created from psychiatric genetic data for use in psychiatric genetic studies. In short, a *psychiatric genetic nosology* seeks to classify patients into categories that correspond to distinct genetic entities. We are not claiming that such a nosology will be useful for clinicians or that it should replace DSM-IV or ICD-10. Our point is simply that psychiatric genetics need not rely on diagnostic constructs created for other purposes.

To be successful, a psychiatric genetic nosology should address the key measurement issues in psychiatric genetics. Each of these issues, in different guises, confronts the problem of diagnostic accuracy. We use the word "accuracy" to indicate the degree to which a diagnosis correctly classifies people with and without a disorder associated with specific susceptibility genes.

> **Key Point:** Although the ultimate goal of psychiatric genetics is to better understand the causes of mental illness, the descriptive categories created for clinical

use may not be ideal for finding genes. Gene finding
may be facilitated by modifying definitions of illness
or incorporating neurobiologic measures into categories defined for clinical use.

There are two fundamental types of diagnostic inaccuracy: false-
negatives and false-positives. False-negatives occur in two ways. The
most straightforward case is when subjects are diagnosed as being well
when they actually have the disease being studied. The second type of
false-negative is caused by reduced penetrance, which means that not
all carriers of a pathogenic genotype will become ill. Thus, these subjects will be classified as not ill even though they carry the disease gene.

False-positive diagnoses also occur in two ways. First, it is possible
that a subject is incorrectly diagnosed as ill. For instance, in the course
of psychiatric interviews, we frequently are forced to reconstruct past
diagnoses based on vague, retrospective reports. It is possible that reports of past symptoms are wrong, leading to a positive diagnosis
when, in fact, the subject never had the disorder.

The second type of false-positive occurs when we correctly classify a
subject as having a disorder but incorrectly classify the genetic subform
of the disorder. For example, some patients diagnosed as having Alzheimer disease do not have the diagnosis confirmed on autopsy; these correspond to the first definition of a false-positive. Among all patients who
have the disease at autopsy, all will be true-positives for the illness, but
false-positives for all but one subform (e.g., a patient with a chromosome 21 mutation would be a false-positive in studies of the chromosome 14 variant). Thus, there are two types of false-positives and both
make it difficult to detect genes for etiologically heterogeneous disorders. If, using clinical data, we could separate genetic subforms, it would
be easier to find genes in the face of causal heterogeneity.

In summary, a genetic nosology must overcome two levels of diagnostic inaccuracy. At the measurement level, our assessment measures
may incorrectly classify subjects with and without the disorder being
studied. At the genetic level, our diagnoses will misclassify subjects as
having (or not having) the gene being studied. Table 7.1 shows the
eight possible outcomes from these two levels of classification. The
four outcomes emphasized in boldface type are cases in which one
level of analysis results in correct classification but the other level results in misclassification. For example, when we diagnose a non-
diseased gene carrier as ill, this person is a false-positive from the
measurement perspective, but a true-positive from the genetic perspective. In contrast, when we diagnose a diseased gene carrier as ill, that

TABLE 7.1. Measurement/Genetic Level Classification Outcomes

	Diagnostic status			
	Gene carriers		Not gene carriers	
True status	Ill	Well	Ill	Well
Diseased	TP/TP	FN/FN	**TP/FP**	**FN/TN**
Nondiseased	**FP/TP**	**TN/FN**	FP/FP	TN/TN

Note. TP, true positive; FP, false positive; TN, true negative; FN, false negative. Entries indicate measurement/genetic level outcomes. **Boldface type** indicates where one level of analysis results in correct classification but the other level results in misclassification. "True status" indicates if the person actually has the underlying genetic disease of interest. Reprinted from Tsuang, M. T., Faraone, S. V., & Lyons, M. J. (1993). Identification of the phenotype in psychiatric genetics. *European Archives of Psychiatry and Clinical Neuroscience, 243,* 131–142. Copyright 1993 Springer-Verlag New York, Inc. Reprinted by permission.

person is a true-positive from both perspectives. Clearly, overcoming these types of measurement error is one of the challenges for the future of psychiatric genetics.

Toward a Psychiatric Genetic Nosology: Decreasing False-Negatives and False-Positives

Variable expression appears to be a common feature of familial psychiatric disorders. Schizophrenia genes may produce schizoaffective disorder, schizotypal personality, atypical psychotic disorders, and a spectrum of other neuropsychologic and neurophysiologic dysfunctions. The biologic relatives of bipolar patients are at high risk for major depressive and bipolar II disorders. The familial predisposition for panic disorder appears to express itself in childhood anxiety disorders and laboratory measures of inhibited behavior. Obsessive–compulsive disorder and chronic tics are alternate manifestations of Tourette syndrome. The genes for attention-deficit hyperactivity disorder may lead to mood, conduct, or anxiety disorders.

Although additional psychiatric phenotypes may be useful for linkage analyses, it seems unlikely that we will eventually discover one-to-one correspondences between genetically influenced processes in the brain and the clinical phenomena that we observe. Since psychiatric signs and symptoms may well be relatively remote effects of genes, psychiatric genetic studies might prove more fruitful if they focus on more direct measures of brain function. This strategy may be especially useful if more than one gene causes the illness. To paraphrase Dr. Steven Matthysse, minor genes for a psychiatric disorder might be major genes for some index of central nervous system dysfunction. If this is so, then measures of this dysfunction may be extremely useful for linkage analysis.

For example, it has been known for some time that schizophrenic patients find it difficult to filter, or "gate," sensory input from the environment. Thus, several experimental protocols have been used to assess sensory gating. Each presents a conditioning stimulus that is followed by a test stimulus. Unlike normal subjects, the schizophrenic patients cannot filter out, or "gate," the second stimulus.

One means of measuring sensory gating uses auditory evoked potentials assayed by the electroencephalogram (EEG), which measures the brain's electrical activity. When a person is resting in a quiet setting, the EEG plots a horizontal line that shows only minor fluctuations over time. The plot looks like a wavy line with many small hills and valleys. When a brief sound is presented to the patient, the EEG will show a rapid increase, then decrease 50 milliseconds after the sound. This spike in activity is called the "P50 wave." If the sound is presented several times, the P50 spike will get smaller and smaller, indicating that the brain is ignoring the sound. The sound has been filtered out or gated. As a group, schizophrenic patients cannot ignore the sound, so their P50 spike does not diminish with repeated repetitions of the sound. This P50 deficit provides a biologic basis for something clinicians have known for a long time: schizophrenic patients are distractible, that is, they cannot focus their attention in a normal manner.

Twin studies show the P50 deficit to be heritable. It is found in about 50 percent of the relatives of schizophrenic patients, a rate much higher than what is seen in the population at large. Notably, many relatives show the deficit without having schizophrenia. Dr. Robert Freedman and colleagues showed that, in families with multiple cases of schizophrenia, the P50 deficit was linked to a locus near chromosome 15q13-14, the site of the alpha-7 nicotinic receptor, which is one of many receptor types that mediate the transmission of neural signals in the brain.

These investigators have argued that other data also favor a link between schizophrenia and abnormalities in nicotinic receptors. Substances that interfere with nicotinic receptor activity exacerbate some schizophrenia symptoms. Moreover, most schizophrenic patients smoke cigarettes and the nicotine from smoking is known to transiently normalize the P50 deficit among schizophrenic patients. Thus, nicotinic receptor systems appear to regulate sensory gating, suggesting that mutations in this nicotinic receptor gene impair sensory gating and increase the risk for schizophrenia. One remarkable feature of Dr. Freedman's finding is that, although the alpha-7 nicotinic receptor region was linked to the P50 deficit, he could not demonstrate that linkage when he used schizophrenia as the affected phenotype in his analyses. Thus, his results provide concrete evidence that the use of alternative phenotypes can detect genes when the frank disorder cannot.

Alternative phenotypes like the P50 deficit must be used cautiously for two reasons. One problem arises when many phenotypic indicators are available for a single disease. Consider the example of schizophrenia. As we noted in Chapter 3, there are several clinical and neurobiologic measures that reflect the genetic liability to this disorder. When a linkage study collects several of these, it becomes possible to test for linkage using many different definitions of who is and who is not affected. This increases the risk that a positive linkage finding will be due to chance alone. There are statistical solutions to this problem, but each of these solutions is accompanied by some loss in statistical power.

Thus, if linkage analysts are to benefit from phenotypic indicators, these indicators must be used judiciously. One approach to the problem of multiple disease definitions is to define a diagnostic hierarchy prior to linkage analysis. The top level of the hierarchy includes the core definition of the illness, while subsequent lower levels use increasingly broader definitions. For example, a schizophrenia linkage study could include at its top level schizophrenia and schizoaffective disorder, depressed. At the second level, psychotic disorder NOS and schizotypal personality disorder could be added. A third level could add individuals who exhibit neurobiologic abnormalities. The first level minimizes the likelihood of false-positive diagnoses. As lower levels are included, the sensitivity will increase, but the false-positive rate also increases.

A second problem hampers the use of alternative phenotypes: it is possible for such phenotypes to be useless, even though their prevalence among relatives of diseased subjects is statistically greater than their prevalence in the general population. Alternative phenotypes are helpful because they decrease the false-negative rate (i.e., they increase penetrance). However, this decrease in the false-negative rate is usually accompanied by an increase in the false-positive rate (i.e., the phenotypic indicators are usually more prevalent among controls than the disease under study). For example, the rate of oculomotor dysfunction among relatives of schizophrenic patients ranges from 14 to 50 percent. Since this is greater than the 10 percent rate of schizophrenia and related psychoses among relatives, oculomotor dysfunction decreases the false-negative rate. But this ignores a key point: although rates of oculomotor impairment are statistically greater among relatives of schizophrenic patients compared with controls, the rate among controls is two to eight times greater than the 1 percent population risk for schizophrenia. This suggests that the use of oculomotor measures as a phenotypic indicator may increase false-positives.

> **Key Point:** Because most mental illnesses are probably caused by several genes acting together, scientists study simpler, related phenotypes in the hopes that they will have a simpler genetic etiology. As a hypothetical example, if schizophrenia is caused by five genes, scientists may be able to discover five neurobiologic measures each corresponding to one of these genes.

How do we know if the trade-off between false-negatives and false-positives makes a phenotypic indicator more or less useful? Dr. Neil Risch suggested a simple method. He showed that the power of a linkage study is directly related to the ratio of two prevalences: the prevalence among relatives of ill probands and the prevalence in the general population. The greater the ratio, the more power. Thus, one way to increase the statistical power of linkage analysis is to define a phenotype that is highly prevalent among relatives of ill probands but rare in the general population. It follows that an alternative phenotype will be most useful if it increases Risch's prevalence ratio. If it maintains the same ratio, it may be made useful by increasing the number of families informative for linkage analysis. For example, families with two or more cases of schizophrenia are rare; their ascertainment is a difficult, time-consuming, and expensive process. Many more families would be informative if we used alternative phenotypes to designate affection.

Dr. David Greenberg suggested that a phenotype definition strategy used for epilepsy might prove useful for psychiatric illness. For a linkage study, he and his colleagues decide to sample families via a specific type of proband, one with juvenile myoclonic epilepsy (JME). However, since previous research showed that some clinically normal relatives of JME patients had abnormal EEGs, they decided to use JME or the presence of an abnormal EEG to define the affected phenotype among family members. When individuals with abnormal EEGs were classified as affected, the lod score (i.e., the evidence for linkage) was statistically significant at 3.8, nearly quadruple the nonsignificant value obtained when abnormal EEGs were considered unaffected.

Since this positive linkage finding has been independently replicated, we cannot attribute it to the play of chance. As Dr. Greenberg discussed, the implications for psychiatric research are straightforward: select probands using a very circumscribed phenotype, but use a broader definition of phenotypes for family members. For example, a schizophrenia linkage project might select families by starting with probands who have Kraepelinian schizophrenia—which is defined by a five-year history of illness and complete dependence on others. Then the criteria for affection status could be broadened to include other cases of schizophrenia, other disorders, and alternative phenotypes according to a prespecified diagnostic hierarchy.

The official diagnostic nomenclature used by clinicians and most researchers treats diagnoses as discrete, binary entities: the patient is either ill or not ill. In contrast, measurement approaches in the psychologic literature focus on dimensional traits that can take on a range of values. The concept of "caseness" lies between these two extremes. Put simply, *caseness* is a dimensional measure of the degree to which we believe that a subject is truly ill.

Caseness has an intuitive appeal that conforms to the realities of diagnosis that face both clinicians and researchers. Some patients clearly have a disorder; others certainly do not. Many more fall between the extremes of diagnostic clarity. It is sensible to associate each of these uncertain cases with an index of caseness that expresses the probability that he or she truly has the disorder. Although such an index would not necessarily deal with the genetic level of diagnostic error, it should facilitate genetic analyses to the degree that it corresponds to the true (but unobservable) illness status of the subject.

Dr. Jurg Ott showed how any index of caseness can be used in a linkage analysis. His method assumes that subjects are assigned weights indicating the probability that they are affected. These weights can be subjective probability judgments made by diagnosticians, or predictions made by mathematical models of disease expression. In a linkage analysis algorithm, these weights can be used to determine the penetrance of each genotype for diagnoses made with varying degrees of certainty.

One appeal of caseness measures is that they can summarize the multiple sources of diagnostic and neurobiologic data that bear on the definition of psychiatric phenotypes. Instead of conducting several analyses that test linkage to a hierarchy of conditions, each condition can be assigned a weight that indicates the probability that a subject with the condition has the genotype of interest. For example, in a schizophrenia linkage study, a schizophrenic subject might be given a weight of 1, a subject with schizotypal personality and oculomotor dysfunction a weight of .8, and a subject with either schizotypal personality or oculomotor dysfunction a weight of .6.

THE FUTURE OF PREDICTIVE GENETIC TESTING

After reading Chapter 6, you may have been puzzled by the large gap between the theory and practice of psychiatric genetics. On the one hand, we have described molecular genetic technologies capable of defining the chemical basis for the inheritance of mental illness. But on the other hand, when discussing the applications of genetic data to genetic counseling, we did not show how DNA, chromosomes, or any other biological product might facilitate our work.

The reason for this is straightforward: unlike other diseases for which DNA testing has become routine, our knowledge of the molecular genetics of psychiatric disease is too rudimentary for use in genetic counseling. But the future will bring changes. These have been foreshadowed by genetic linkage findings in Alzheimer disease, which suggest that DNA testing may be useful to predict who is and who is not at risk for the disease in families known to be affected by specific genetic forms of the disorder. Because genetic tests for Alzheimer disease and other psychiatric conditions will very likely become routine in the future, this section describes how such tests might be used based on how they are currently used for nonpsychiatric diseases.

Presymptomatic Genetic Testing

Table 7.2 lists some diseases for which genetic tests are currently available. Many of the tests are used to confirm clinical diagnoses but most can also be used for testing presymptomatic individuals or for prenatal diagnosis. However, guidelines established by the American Society of Human Genetics strongly discourage presymptomatic testing for adult-onset conditions in at-risk children under 18 who are asymptomatic due to the potential adverse psychological and emotional effects such information could have on these children and their parents.

Scientists discover genes and pathogenic mutations on a weekly basis. These discoveries, however, must await more extensive studies in families at risk before they become clinically useful. Before clinical tests

TABLE 7.2. Examples of Diseases Having Commercially Available Genetic Tests for Presymptomatic or Prenatal Testing

Alpha thalassemia	Kennedy disease
Breast cancer	Myotonic dystrophy
Cystic fibrosis	Sickle cell anemia
Epidermolysis bullosa simplex	Spinocerebellar ataxia type, 1
Fragile-X mental retardation	Spinocerebellar ataxia type, 3
Huntington disease	

can be developed, we need detailed information about the pathogenic mutation, for example, its frequency in the population, its penetrance among gene carriers, and its frequency among those with the disease. Without such data we cannot readily use and interpret test results.

Consider this example. Scientists have discovered two genes associated with breast cancer: BRCA1 and BRCA2. Intensive studies of these genes have found over 140 different mutations. Does this mean that genetic tests will be able to find all or most women who are at high risk for breast cancer? Sadly, the answer is no. Only about 5 to 10 percent of breast cancers have a strong genetic component, and these two genes account for about 50 to 80 percent of these cases. These facts have led to DNA testing guidelines for breast cancer that preclude screening in the general population, but recommend it for the small fraction of women who are at especially high risk for mutations in the two breast cancer genes.

The risk for carrying a breast cancer gene mutation is greatest for women who have a family history of breast cancer, especially when the affected family member had the disease earlier than age 50, or had cancer in both breasts. The level of risk also rises with the presence of multiple relatives in more than one generation who have had breast or ovarian cancer. For families that meet the above criteria, testing can be done either to establish the mutation status of the person with breast or ovarian cancer or to establish the genetic status of presymptomatic consultands with mutation-positive relatives.

As you can see, the availability of known mutations provides genetic counselors with precise information for making predictions about illness onset in presymptomatic family members. Nevertheless, even in such cases, we sometimes cannot predict outcomes with certainty. For example, breast cancer is not 100 percent penetrant in BRCA1 gene carriers; they have an 80 percent chance of developing breast cancer by age 65. Therefore, even when DNA tests are available, the ultimate outcome of the consultand may not be known with certainty.

Adding to this uncertainty are technical limitations. Commercially available genetic tests for breast cancer only screen for the most common mutations. Issues of cost and feasibility make it impossible to design a cost-effective clinical test that screens for all known mutations. That would simply be too expensive. Therefore, only positive results from breast cancer testing are completely informative. Negative results indicate the absence of common mutations but they cannot rule out the presence of rare mutations.

> **Key Point:** Presymptomatic predictive genetic testing is currently not available for psychiatric disorders. Such

> testing will not be available until research proves it to
> have clinical value and society has grappled with the
> ethical issues it raises.

Alzheimer disease provides a neuropsychiatric example of a disease for which genetic testing may be available for a small minority of individuals. As previously discussed, scientists have identified three genes that cause early-onset Alzheimer disease in families that show a pattern of autosomal dominant transmission. The gene known as presenilin-2 is on chromosome 1, presenilin-1 is on chromosome 14, and the amyloid precursor protein gene is on chromosome 21. Although the discovery of these genes was extremely important to the understanding of the pathogenesis of Alzheimer disease, clear autosomal dominant transmission is seen in less than 1 percent of all cases of Alzheimer disease. Today, presymptomatic testing is available on a research basis but it is only relevant to individuals from these high-risk families.

Eventually, the mutations in Alzheimer disease genes may be used in clinical practice. For example, imagine a genetic counselor presented with a 25-year-old client who has a family history of Alzheimer disease in two prior generations, suggesting autosomal dominant transmission. If we observe a mutation in an affected relative, then the absence of the mutation in the client would indicate minimal risk for early-onset Alzheimer disease. Conversely, the presence of the mutation in the client would suggest high risk. We would not put this risk at 100 percent until the penetrance of these mutations are known with certainty.

Risk prediction from genetic tests is more difficult for the more common form of Alzheimer disease, which onsets after age 65, and has a complex mode of inheritance. Like other complex psychiatric disorders, it is likely that most late-onset Alzheimer disease cases are caused by the joint effects of many genes along with environmental factors. As we described in Chapter 5, Dr. Allen Roses and colleagues have already found one gene that increases the risk for late-onset Alzheimer disease: the apolipoprotein E (APOE) gene on chromosome 19.

People who have two copies of the ε4 variant of this gene are at a much higher risk for developing Alzheimer disease, but many who are in this group will not develop Alzheimer disease and many patients with Alzheimer disease do not have the genotype. As a result, the APOE gene is not clinically useful for genetic counseling. Thus, the American Society of Human Genetics currently does not recommend APOE testing for either routine clinical diagnosis or for predictive testing. This recommendation does not challenge the widely held belief that APOE makes one susceptible to Alzheimer disease. In fact, the society's report suggested that a greater utility for APOE genotyping might emerge in the evaluation of treatment options for individual patients. However, until more clinical research is completed, there is no compelling evidence supporting its routine use.

Lessons from Predictive Testing in Huntington Disease

Because Huntington disease was the first neuropsychiatric disorder for which genetic testing became available, it is a useful prototype for illustrating the clinical issues raised by predictive DNA testing. Two methods of DNA testing are available for Huntington disease. After the initial report of genetic linkage in 1983, the implicated genetic region was narrowed down to a region containing 10 million base-pairs. This was small enough to permit indirect mutation testing using genetic markers that were closely linked to the Huntington disease gene. This type of testing defines at-risk individuals (i.e., relatives of Huntington disease patients) as being at low, moderate, or high risk for carrying the Huntington disease gene.

After the Huntington disease gene was physically identified and sequenced in 1993, direct mutation testing became available. This is the preferred and standard method of testing since it directly detects the Huntington disease mutation. Thus, consultands can be 98 to 99 percent confident of their results. Although this high level of certainty is, from a purely logical point of view, a strength of direct DNA testing, we must be concerned about the potential harm of such news to recipients.

Experience with Huntington disease shows that genetic counselors must be prepared to handle a wide range of psychologic and emotional reactions to genetic testing. Candidates for DNA testing will arrive with preconceptions about what testing might tell them and what the implications of that information might be. Understanding the consultand's baseline expectations and emotional state is a precondition for sensitively guiding him or her through the testing process.

After undergoing pretest counseling and the blood draw to provide DNA, some consultands may become very emotional. For them, this is a time of heightened uncertainty and apprehension. They may suffer from anxiety, depression, or even suicidal ideation. Some consultands will seek to terminate the testing process, others will forge on. For individuals in both groups, it is essential that such decisions derive not from the impulse of emotion, but from the guidance of reason. Some consultands may be so wrought up over the testing process that they will require mental health treatment before proceeding.

Informing consultands that they will, with nearly 100 percent certainty, develop Huntington disease (or any other serious disease) is not an easy process for either the counselor or the consultand. Regardless of whether the news is good or bad, you should advise consultands to bring a supportive relative to the session during which you will communicate the results of DNA testing. For obvious reasons, consultands often show extreme emotional reactions upon learning that they have the Huntington disease gene. Because most people who seek testing come from high-risk families, they have witnessed close relatives suffer a slow and progressively disabling death. They have every reason to feel utter despair and to become clinically depressed. Such consultands will need to be closely followed to monitor adverse effects and help them cope with their impending disability and death.

Other consultands will accept their genetic fate with equanimity. Having already steeled themselves for the worst, they may view the results as confirming a long suspected fact. Such consultands may feel relieved that they can finally plan their lives accordingly. They may find subsequent sessions useful to facilitate planning, to help them cope with the reactions of relatives, and to prevent or mitigate any adverse reactions that might emerge.

Consultands who learn that they are not at genetic risk have much to celebrate. Having won the "genetic lottery," they can now plan how to spend the additional years of life they have been awarded. But even with such genetic "winners" there is need for clinical caution. Initial euphoria may give way to sorrow and suffering. Some consultands will develop survival guilt, feeling acutely the loss of departed family members and the anguish of those known to carry the gene. Others may lose a sense of personal identity that once had been molded by a vision of life cut short by a heritable condition. They may have attributed problems in their life to having the "family disease" and will be frustrated to learn that their problems remain when they are freed from that fate. Extended posttest psychotherapy may be indicated for these individuals, as they are at risk for psychopathology and psychosocial dysfunction.

Although Huntington disease provides a useful illustration of DNA testing and its potential impact on consultands, we must emphasize the many differences that exist between Huntington disease and most psychiatric conditions. Huntington disease is caused by a single autosomal dominant gene; therefore, an offspring is at a 50 percent risk for inheriting the gene. This differs from most psychiatric conditions, which are probably multifactorial and definitely pose a much lower risk to relatives. Almost all individuals who carry the Huntington disease gene develop the disease by age 80. In other words, it is completely penetrant. By contrast, most psychiatric disorders are incompletely penetrant: they do not occur in all people who carry the pathogenic genotype.

Furthermore, the gene disrupted in Huntington disease is the same in all affected individuals as is the nature of the mutation: individuals with a trinucleotide repeat size greater than 37 are considered to have inherited the gene. Thus, there is no ambiguity created by genetic heterogeneity, which is likely for psychiatric conditions. For example, there are many different mutations in the presenilin-1 gene on chromosome 14 that cause one type of familial Alzheimer disease. Screening for all these mutations is extremely labor-intensive and not practical for routine genetic counseling. In addition, when many mutations are possible, failure to find a specific one may provide a false sense of security.

On a positive note, when presymptomatic genetic testing of psychiatric conditions becomes available, it will in many cases have useful clinical applications beyond genetic counseling. Unlike Huntington disease, which is currently incurable, we do have effective treatments for many psychiatric conditions. The effectiveness of current treatments suggests that preventive treatments might work once we identify people at high genetic risk and have a lucid understanding of the mechanisms of gene action. In this light, presymptomatic identification of genetically susceptible individuals would allow earlier intervention prior to the development of potentially debilitating psychiatric symptoms.

Despite the potential uses of presymptomatic testing for psychiatric disease, such testing is currently not possible and should not be used until scientists demonstrate that it has clinical value. Drs. Gilbert Welch and Wylie Burke described four uncertainties about the genetic testing of chronic genetically complex diseases like psychiatric illness. The major problem to be faced by psychiatric genetics will be the inability to predict with certainty who will become ill, even after specific disease genes are discovered. Recall that twin studies show that many people who are genetically identical to a schizophrenic patient will not themselves develop schizophrenia. The same could be said of bipolar disorder, major depression, and most other psychiatric conditions. Given this fact of complex inheritance, it seems likely that, even after the genes for these disorders have been catalogued, even knowledge of who carries these genes will not allow us to predict who will develop the disorders with certainty.

Even if risk prediction is uncertain, one might argue that the ability to describe the probability of illness will be useful. But can we be certain about the accuracy of such probabilities? In theory, we could use extensive research to compute accurate probabilities. In practice, such computations might not be feasible. Notably, most initial genetic studies focus on mutations in high-risk families that have many affected members. But, in addition to harboring the mutation, these families may differ from the population at large in other ways. For example, they may have been exposed to environmental toxins or they may harbor another unknown mutation that is needed to activate the known mutation. Due to these potential differences, the predictive validity of the mutations found in high-risk families may not be relevant to the general population. Thus, before they can be used for presymptomatic testing in the general population, the predictive validity of proposed tests must be tested in that population. This will be very costly and perhaps not feasible when, as is the case for the BRCA1 breast cancer gene, over 500 different mutations have been found.

The third uncertainty described by Drs. Welch and Burke is the uncertainty about the right age for testing. Even if we had a valid genetic test for Alzheimer disease, should we use it to assess the risk status of schoolchildren? Of young adults? Of older adults? Screening people for diseases that will onset in the distant future places a huge psychological burden on those found to be gene carriers. Such information has the potential to diminish self-esteem, create a sense of hopelessness, trigger depression, and disrupt family relationships. Thus, information about genetic risks for complex disease should be given at the age research shows is best for the well-being of the person being tested. Presumably, the timing of these genetic tests would be tied to our knowledge of when is the best time to intervene with preventive treatments. But this itself is the fourth area of uncertainty: the value of preventive treatments.

> **Key Point:** Presymptomatic testing for psychiatric disorders will not be clinically meaningful until we can be certain about (1) who is at risk for specific disorders, (2) the accuracy of risk prediction, (3) the best time to provide test results, and (4) how to use genetic test data to improve the lives of those being tested.

In an ideal world, presymptomatic genetic testing would improve the outcome of the minority of screened persons found to harbor disease genes. For example, if someday we could assay the set of genes that predispose to psychosis, we would be able to monitor adolescents at very high-risk for psychosis. Close surveillance of these high risk adolescents would lead to the very early treatment of emergent psychoses and a better overall outcome. Moreover, if preventive treatment protocols were developed and tested, early identification of high-risk adolescents might perhaps prevent psychosis. Under these ideal but hypothetical conditions, genetic testing for psychosis genes would be warranted. It will, however, require much research subsequent to the discovery of such genes before we will know if preventive programs will have any value.

For some psychiatric disorders, it is possible that the four uncertainties described by Drs. Welch and Burke will be clarified by research. But that work will take many years—if not decades—to accomplish. Before it is completed, it will be difficult to justify presymptomatic genetic testing for mental illness.

THE FUTURE OF MENTAL HEALTH TREATMENT

Currently, treatment regimes for most psychiatric disorders are multimodal, relying on both medication and psychosocial therapies to achieve the optimum outcome for patients. Genetic data are unlikely to change this overall approach to treatment, but they will have implications for creating preventive interventions and implementing medical interventions targeted at specific genetic defects.

Early Identification and Prevention of Disorders

A national consensus of scientists and clinicians supports the adage that an ounce of prevention is worth a pound of cure. The rationale for prevention can be easily seen by referring to the theoretical model we presented in Figure 1.2 (refer back to p. 9 in Chapter 1). The figure shows three levels of disease manifestation: a neurodevelopmental prodrome, the onset of frank psychopathology, and degeneration into chronic illness.

We will refer to the figure to illustrate two distinctions made in the prevention literature: primary versus secondary prevention and universal preventive interventions versus selective preventive interventions. *Primary prevention* refers to any intervention that stops the onset of disease. For example, we can prevent or delay heart disease by not smoking, reducing cholesterol intake, and exercising frequently. There is no simple formula of this sort for mental illness, but we can imagine how prevention might be possible in the future.

As Figure 1.2 suggests, primary prevention protocols could operate on two levels. First, they could block early environmental insults and prevent neurodevelopmental abnormalities and subsequent illness. For example, improving the pre-, peri-, and postnatal care of children born to schizophrenic mothers might limit the impact of genes and spare children from both schizophrenia and its neurodevelopmental precursors. Primary prevention protocols could also block later environmental insults to prevent the onset of psychopathology but not the earlier onset neurodevelopmental abnormalities. For example, having identified an adolescent who exhibits the neuropsychologic and social dysfunction that are schizophrenia's neurodevelopmental precursors, we might use a family therapy program to help the child avoid overstimulating environments that might trigger psychosis. Or, once the biologic underpinnings of psychosis are understood, scientists might be able to create a drug that prevents psychosis in these vulnerable adolescents.

Unlike primary prevention, *secondary prevention* does not prevent illness; instead, it mitigates its course. For the case of schizophrenia, it seems that psychosis is harmful to the brain. Each episode weakens the brain, making the patient more susceptible to subsequent episodes and increasing the likelihood of chronic symptoms. Thus, treatment early in the course of illness is believed to lessen chronicity and improve the course of illness compared with treatment later in the course of illness. This reality has motivated the development of secondary prevention programs that attempt to identify and treat people with schizophrenia as soon as possible subsequent to the first onset of psychosis.

In addition to considering what stage of the disease process is appropriate for intervention, prevention protocols distinguish two types of target populations. *Selective preventive programs* focus intervention resources on individuals whose risk of developing mental illness is significantly higher than average. For example, because children with conduct disorder are known to be at high risk for substance abuse, they would be a logical group to target for a selective preventive program for substance abuse.

> **Key Point:** Psychiatric genetic data may eventually allow us to create selective prevention programs aimed at helping people known to be at high genetic risk for specific disorders.

In contrast to selective interventions, *universal preventive programs* apply prevention resources to all members of a designated population without regard for high-risk status. Such programs are usually implemented in community settings such as schools. For example, the Drug Abuse Resistance Education (DARE) program has been used to prevent drug use by all students in schools that have accepted the program. When a school sets up a DARE program, all its enrolled children are involved. The intervention does not target a group believed to be at highest risk.

The discovery of specific genes for mental illness will allow us to select a subset of children who are at risk for subsequent onsets of mental illness. Thus, such data will lead to selective, primary preventive interventions. Currently, it is not possible to either design or implement such interventions because we have yet to discover genes that will allow us to predict with certainty who will and who will not become mentally ill. But imagine what might be possible in the future. Genetic diagnostic protocols may someday tell parents the genetic strengths and weaknesses of their offspring. If so, preventive services to stop, mitigate, or delay the onset of psychopathology could be offered to high-risk children.

These preventive services could be either psychosocial or medical. *Psychosocial prevention programs* would seek to create environments that prevent genes from exerting their pathogenic effects. These programs might change the social learning regimes of children or modulate their exposure to stress. *Medical treatment programs* might use medications that target the effects of aberrant genes. They might even attempt to change the gene itself through gene therapy, which we discuss later in this chapter.

> **Key Point:** The use of genetic data to select people for prevention protocols does not require us to limit our study to the efficacy of putative biologic preventive treatments. The use of psychosocial interventions to modify the environment or the coping strategies of at risk people should also be studied.

To move genetically based prevention protocols from the realm of the imaginary world to that of the real world, we would need to establish at least two facts: (1) that it is possible to accurately define a population at risk for a disorder and (2) that there is a compelling rationale for any proposed preventive treatment. To help you understand how complex these issues are, we will discuss them in the context of two examples: schizophrenic and anxiety disorders.

Childhood Predictors of Schizophrenic Disorders

We have said that genetically based primary prevention programs will be *selective*; that is, they will identify and treat the subset of children at highest risk for a disorder, for example, schizophrenia. You might ask:

Why wait for the discovery of genes? Can't we simply apply a program to all schoolchildren? Because a universal program would be sure to target *all* future schizophrenic patients, wouldn't it be very effective? This line of reasoning seems compelling, but it has a fatal flaw: it fails to consider the costs of treating children who will not become schizophrenic.

Let's consider a hypothetical school-based intervention for schizophrenia. Epidemiologic studies indicate that a school of 1,000 children will have among its students only 10 who will eventually develop a schizophrenic disorder. Thus, if we applied a prevention program to all the children in the school, we would unnecessarily treat 990 children and correctly treat 10. This would not be a problem if the prevention program was very inexpensive and had no adverse effects. But that is not realistic. A prevention program for schizophrenia would likely be very expensive and may well have adverse effects. Thus, we need some method for selecting specific children for the preventive intervention.

One possibility would be to choose adolescent children or siblings of schizophrenic patients. We know from genetic studies that this group has a tenfold elevated risk for psychosis and is entering the age period of greatest risk for its onset. This approach is better than selecting all children but it still falls short: only 10 percent of the selected group would develop schizophrenia or a related psychotic disorder. Thus, for every 1,000 adolescents selected for treatment, 100 would need the treatment and 900 would not need the treatment. Even if the treatment were 100 percent effective for the 100 at-risk teens, it would be difficult to justify treating the 900 who are not at risk.

Following the logic of Figure 1.2, one method of further improving our definition of "high risk for schizophrenia" would be to select children who show signs of the neurodevelopmental brain abnormalities believed to precede schizophrenia. We discussed these in Chapter 3, as spectrum conditions, psychopathologic features, personality traits, or measures of brain dysfunction believed to reflect the genetic predisposition to a disorder.

Fortunately, research suggests that some spectrum conditions may improve risk prediction to the level where they would prove useful in defining populations at very high risk for schizophrenia. For example, several groups of investigators have shown that neuromotor abnormalities and attentional deficits in childhood predict subsequent schizophrenia or related disorders later in life.

Also, consider the results of a retrospective study by Drs. Elaine Walker and Richard Lewine. They collected videotapes of schizophrenic patients that had been made in childhood, prior to the onset of the patients' schizophrenia. They then asked expert clinicians to examine these videos, as well as videos of children who did not become schizophrenic. Although these clinicians made some errors, they were able to separate most of the preschizophrenic children from the normal children. The former children showed poorer fine and gross motor coordination, poorer eye contact, more negative affect, and diminished social responsiveness.

Although these and other studies are well on the way to developing a reasonably accurate ability to predict who will develop schizophrenia, primary prevention studies also need a compelling rationale to support an attempt at preventive treatment. Theoretically, psychosocial interventions could choose two foci for intervention: children "at risk" and their environments. Such interventions might help high-risk children withstand common stresses that may be toxic to people predisposed to schizophrenia.

Clearly, further research is needed to create a scientific foundation for preventive psychosocial interventions for schizophrenia. In addition, the possibility that psychopharmacologic approaches might improve the stress tolerance of high-risk children should also be considered.

Behavioral Inhibition to the Unfamiliar and Anxiety Disorders

Even a casual observer of children will soon realize that some are shy and withdrawn, clinging to their parents, sitting quietly in classrooms, and not participating in peer activities. Are these shy children passing through a developmental phase soon to be eclipsed by a growing repertoire of social behaviors? Or will they struggle throughout life with social anxiety, difficult relationships, and, perhaps, frank anxiety disorders?

Behavioral inhibition appears to be a somewhat enduring trait. For example, Dr. Jerome Kagan's research group at Harvard University defined a group of two year olds as either behaviorally inhibited or uninhibited when exposed to unfamiliar settings, people, and objects. They examined these children again at ages four, five, and seven. The children who had been inhibited at age two tended to remain inhibited, while those who had been uninhibited tended to remain uninhibited. To examine shy children, Dr. Kagan created a laboratory-based measure of childhood temperament called "behavioral inhibition to the unfamiliar." Dr. Kagan and colleagues reported that 15 to 20 percent of children show behavioral inhibition. Behaviorally inhibited children consistently display fear and withdrawal in situations that are novel or unfamiliar. These children are irritable as infants, shy and fearful as toddlers, and cautious, quiet, and introverted when they reach school age. In contrast, 25 to 30 percent of children are uninhibited. They socialize easily, are bold and gregarious, and not upset by novel situations. Because most children lie between these extremes, behavioral inhibition is best considered as a quantitative dimension of temperament varying from extreme inhibition to extreme lack of inhibition.

Behavioral inhibition also has physiologic manifestations. Inhibited infants show greater sympathetic tone in the cardiovascular system, have higher fetal heart rates a few weeks before birth, and also have higher heart rates at two weeks of age. Older inhibited children have higher and more stable heart rates, and show an acceleration of heart rate and pupillary dilation when faced with mild psychologic stress. Furthermore, in middle childhood, inhibited children show a greater increase in diastolic blood pressure when their posture changes from a sitting to a standing position, suggesting increased noradrenergic tone.

These physiologic data imply a more reactive sympathetic influence on cardiovascular functioning in inhibited children. Dr. Kagan has theorized that inhibited children have a low threshold for arousal in the brain's limbic system, especially when exposed to unfamiliar events. As a result, these children show abnormally high levels of sympathetic activation in the peripheral nervous system. This excessive activation presumably leads to shyness and other types of inhibited behavior.

These studies of behavioral inhibition had been conducted to study childhood temperament, not psychopathology. Yet Dr. Kagan's descriptions of inhibited children at school age were strikingly similar to clinical descriptions of children of agoraphobic patients. They also mirrored how agoraphobic adults had described their own childhoods. For example, inhibited children tended to be fearful during the first days of school; they also showed marked signs of separation anxiety and avoidance. These clinical features, along with evidence of increased physiologic arousal, suggested that measures developed to assess behavioral inhibition might be early identifiers of anxiety-proneness in young children.

Because of the behavioral and physiologic correspondences between behavioral inhibition and anxiety disorders, Drs. Jerrold Rosenbaum and Joseph Biederman, of the Massachusetts General Hospital and Harvard Medical School, began a study of behavioral inhibition among young children whose parents had panic disorder and agoraphobia. This research team found a higher risk for behavioral inhibition among the children of panic-disordered parents compared with children of parents without panic disorder. They also found behavioral inhibition to predict an increased risk for anxiety disorders in children three years later. This line of research suggests that behavioral inhibition may be a precursor to panic, and perhaps to other anxiety disorders. If future work confirms these findings, it may be possible to use behavioral inhibition to select children for anxiety prevention programs.

Medical Interventions for Genetic Defects

Consider this extraordinary fact: although decades of research have unearthed the biologic roots of mental illness, much of the evidence, albeit compelling, is circumstantial, indirect, inconclusive. In the detective work that is science we have found few "smoking guns." But when specific genes for specific illnesses are found this ambiguity will lessen. We will finally be able to identify mutant genes, show that they produce aberrant proteins, and determine how their interactions with the environment and other genes lead to mental illness. This comprehension of causal mechanisms will allow scientists to develop medical interventions targeted at specific genetic defects.

To illustrate some possibilities, consider two strategies for treating genetic disorders: correcting the primary biochemical defects caused by defective genes and replacing or modifying defective genes. In some cases, correcting the primary biochemical deficit requires an environmental change. The treatment can be as simple as avoiding certain foods. Phenylketonuria (PKU) is an autosomal recessive condition that prevents metabolism of phenylalanine. Its treatment is straightforward: eliminate phenylalanine from the diet. Such a diet prevents mental retardation, seizures, and behavioral symptoms such as hyperactivity, distractibility, and irritability. Another example is reduction of cholesterol intake in persons with hereditary forms of hypercholesterolemia, to reduce the risk of atherosclerotic heart disease. Alternatively, affected people can take drugs designed to reduce cholesterol levels. Physicians can correct some biochemical defects by supplementing patients with a missing protein. For example, persons with hemophilia can achieve near normal blood clotting capacity by receiving supplements of the natural blood clotting factor disrupted by their genetic defect.

Today, clinicians routinely correct genetically caused biochemical defects by modifying the environment or supplementing patients with missing proteins. In contrast, gene therapy is a novel, developing technology rarely used in clinical settings. *Gene therapy* refers to a class of procedures that remove mutant genes from cells and replace them with normal versions. Even in our era of laser-guided microsurgery, the molecular surgery of genes sounds preposterous. But it is not.

Gene therapy made its debut in 1990 when scientists and physicians at the National Institutes of Health (NIH) treated a girl (we'll call her Sara) suffering from severe combined immune deficiency (SCID), which leaves its victims vulnerable to massive, lethal infections from common diseases. Without treatment, Sara would have suffered a grim fate: children with SCID are usually attacked by overwhelming infections and rarely survive to adulthood. For Sara, even a common childhood illness like chicken pox could be life-threatening. This fatal disease has a genetic source: a mutant gene creates white blood cells that are not capable of mounting an effective counterattack to infection.

Prior to gene therapy, the only treatment for SCID was avoidance of contact with pathogens. This approach to disease management required patients to live in sterile conditions, an expensive process that also severely limited the patient's ability to interact with parents and peers. Fortunately, NIH researchers realized that the genetic source of SCID might also harbor a medical solution. They reasoned that if they could modify Sara's white blood cells by inserting the missing piece of DNA, her cells would function normally to fight infection.

As you can imagine, this is a complicated process. First, the doctors had to remove white blood cells from Sara. Then these cells were genetically modified and returned to Sara's blood stream. Any errors in this process would weaken the treatment, and possibly harm Sara. After refining the methodology, the research team collected Sara's blood and completed the experiment. All were pleased to learn that her new white blood cells were functioning normally. Sara's immune system was strengthened and she became more resistant to infection. Unfortunately, the new white blood cells die after a few months. Thus, frequent treatments are needed.

> **Key Point:** Gene therapy sounds like science fiction but it has already had some successes and is currently being studied for hundreds of diseases. It has, however, not been used for a disease with a complex mode of inheritance. We cannot be certain if the method will be applicable to the genes that cause mental illness.

Since the groundbreaking gene therapy of SCID, more than 200 human gene therapy protocols have been approved for research and over 2,000 patients have received experimental gene therapy. However, only a handful of patients have benefited from this form of treatment. We will discuss two examples: cancer and cystic fibrosis.

Most cancer clinical trials have targeted the destruction of cancer cells. One strategy involves drug susceptibility genes. Cells that contain such genes will die when exposed to a specific drug. Cancer scientists reasoned that if such genes could be inserted into cancer cells, they could be selectively killed by administering the drug. Moreover, when the cancer cells replicate, the new copies retain the drug-sensitive gene so they too can be selectively killed. In another strategy, the body's immune system is changed to enhance the recognition and destruction of tumor cells. So far, success has been limited due to the inability to properly regulate gene expression as well as the inability to deliver a sufficient quantity of the gene into the target cells.

Gene therapy has also been attempted for cystic fibrosis. In this condition, the affected individual has two copies of the abnormal gene and cannot produce enzymes needed for thinning body secretions. This leads to poor absorption of food in the intestine and infection in the lungs. Gene therapy has attempted to deliver the normal gene to the lungs, so as to promote normal lung function.

Many scientific advances have assisted gene therapy in its transformation from science fiction to science fact. Chief among these was the discovery of methods for transferring DNA into human cells. Because cells are small and genes even smaller, conventional surgical techniques cannot be used. Ironically, the solution to the gene transfer problem was a well-known cause of disease: the virus.

Viruses are simple creatures. Each consists of a DNA core wearing a protein "jacket." The jacket serves as a biological hypodermic syringe that injects viral DNA into the nuclei of unsuspecting cells. This allows the viral DNA to combine with the host cell's DNA and thereby reproduce itself using the cell's reproductive machinery. In doing so viruses cause diseases as mild as the common cold and as severe as AIDS. Despite its bad reputation, the virus has been essential to the development of gene therapy. By replacing viral DNA with human DNA, scientists use the virus as a handy tool that inserts working genes into cells that have defective ones.

For gene therapy to work we need to know which gene is needed and which cells are affected by the disease. In the case of SCID, the mutant gene was known and the white blood cell was identified as the cell in which gene malfunction caused disease. Successful gene therapy also requires that we be able to insert the gene into a sufficient number of cells for the new gene to exert a therapeutic effect. These requirements for gene therapy have created new challenges for a generation of scientists who promise to make molecular medicine a standard tool for the physician of the future.

ETHICAL ISSUES FOR THE SCIENCE AND PRACTICE
OF PSYCHIATRIC GENETICS

There is, perhaps, only one fact that is certain about the future of psychiatric genetics: it will continue to raise ethical challenges for scientists, research participants, clinicians, and patients. Although ethical issues are of concern to everyone in all branches of psychiatry and genetics, they are especially salient for those in psychiatric genetics. This is due to the fact that psychiatry deals with thoughts, emotions, and behavior, the core features that define our selves. Some people are disturbed by the idea that modifying genes could modify these features. They argue that tinkering with the psychologic and emotional machinery of humanity by changing our genetic heritage is akin to playing God. They fear that the potential outcomes, known and unknown, could be devastating.

Science creates knowledge. From an ethical or moral perspective, knowledge is neutral. It is the application of knowledge that brings us into the moral realm. We have seen in our lifetime how the discovery of atomic energy generated tremendous scientific breakthroughs and positive technological achievements. Yet it also pushed humanity to the brink of annihilation. Likewise, the data generated by the Human Genome Project are morally neutral, but the potential applications of this information are not.

Although these issues are enough to alert thoughtful people to the need for ethical inquiry, that quest is further motivated by historical precedent. In its formative years, findings from psychiatric genetics were abused by scientists and politicians to kill rather than to cure. Thus, it is worthwhile to contemplate a short lesson from history as we consider the ethical implications of psychiatric genetic research.

The Shadow of Eugenics

In 1883, the term "eugenics" was coined by the British scientist Francis Galton. This word comes from the Greek terms *eu* (meaning "well") and *genos* (meaning "born"). Galton and many of his contemporaries in Europe and the United States believed that progress had freed mankind from the Darwinian shackles of natural selection. In their view, people who were genetically unfit might now be saved by medicine and would thus live to reproduce and pass their mutant genes to future generations. According to the eugenicists, freedom from natural selection would increase the gene frequency of deleterious genes and thereby pollute the human gene pool.

Eugenics was intended to replace natural selection with an artificial method of selection that would select people with "good" genes for reproduction and discourage those with "bad" ones from transmitting them to offspring. Galton and colleagues argued that eugenics, if successfully applied, would hasten the development of favorable human traits and eliminate those that were harmful to individuals and society.

In Galton's time, support for eugenics was strong enough to prompt the creation of a Eugenics Society, which published its own journal, the *Eugenics Review*. Over the next 50 years, the eugenics movement grew in strength. By 1935, more than half of the states in the United States and several European countries had approved laws allowing the sterilization of "defective" people. Eugenics had become social policy.

Although many were convinced by the cold logic of the eugenics movement, others voiced dissent. Behaviorists and other social scientists argued that eugenics policies were not adequately informed about the role of environmental agents in causing disease and disability. From an ethical perspective, critics of eugenics argued that all people had an unalienable right to reproduce, a right that could not be taken away from the mentally retarded, the physically handicapped, the mentally ill, the medically infirm or any other human being.

Others decried eugenics laws for dictating personal and social values. In this view, eugenics provided a pseudoscientific veneer for policies intended to promulgate racial, ethnic, or class prejudices. Moreover, from the anti-eugenics perspective there was a fine line between decreeing who should and who should not reproduce and deciding who should and who should not be alive. If eugenicists were willing to prevent reproduction through sterilization, would they further that goal through extermination?

To many scientists and politicians of the early 1930s, these voices of dissent seemed foolish. But they were prophetic. In the mid-1930s Adolph Hitler and his Nazi regime began a systematic program first to sterilize and then to kill "genetically defective" people. These included the deaf, the blind, the mentally ill, the mute, the mentally retarded, the physically handicapped, and homosexuals. Although accurate estimates are not available, historians believe that Nazi doctors sterilized at least 400,000 people and killed about 100,000.

Key Point: In the first half of the 20th century, eugenics—the idea that public policy could clean up the gene pool—was promoted by scientists in many "developed" countries. In the hands of the Nazis, these ideas led to forced sterilization and wholesale murder.

Prior to the rise of Hitler, German psychiatric genetics had made great strides in demonstrating that genes played a role in causing mental illness. Contemporary researchers in psychiatric genetics are especially disturbed to learn that the Nazis used this research to justify their eugenics policies regarding the mentally ill and that some scientists participated in this corruption of knowledge. Although the extent of medical eugenics killings was small in contrast to the mass murder of the Holocaust, both were driven by the deranged belief that some higher political power could and should separate the genetically defective from the genetically robust. This misuse of genetic data sends an unambiguous warning to contemporary scientists and clinical geneticists. Although the clinical application of genetic data may save lives and diminish disability, its political application could be devastating.

Fortunately, the Nazi abuses of psychiatric genetics contrast sharply to the subsequent development of the field throughout the world. In addition to broadening the scope of knowledge about genetic contributions to mental illness, geneticists have addressed the growing list of ethical and legal issues that this knowledge has created. Notably, by establishing an Ethical, Legal, and Social Initiative (ELSI), the NIH's Human Genome Project has committed substantial resources to address these concerns. Although genetics researchers can participate in ELSI projects, ELSI researchers are not simply geneticists monitoring their own work. Instead, they come from a wide variety of disciplines (e.g., philosophy, law, sociology, genetic counseling), and thus serve as watchdogs for the genetics community.

ELSI researchers have been creating an empirical and intellectual framework, and legislators have been drafting guidelines and statutes to govern the use of genetic information. These researchers are asking many questions: How will genetic data affect the practice of medicine? How will genomics be used in genetic counseling and reproductive decision making? Will genetic data about adoptees be given to potential adoptive parents? Should legislation protect the privacy of genetic information? Should such information be used to gauge insurability or employability? Will the eventual cataloguing of genes influencing thought, behavior, and emotions lead some to adopt a naïve reductionism that equates the essence of humanity with the nucleotide sequences separating us from other organisms? Will a reductionist view of human behavior divert resources to biologic research at the expense of studies aimed at finding psychosocial influences on disease?

Key Point: ELSI is the Ethical, Legal, and Social Initiative of the Human Genome Project. ELSI researchers are the ethical gadflys and watchdogs of the genetics research community. They teach scientists about the ethical pitfalls of the past and will help them avoid those that await them in the future.

Researchers and clinicians involved with psychiatric genetics must consider these questions, listen to the answers, and participate in the formulation and implementation of ethical principles that are sensible for mental illness. That will allow us to unravel the mysteries of mental illness while doing no harm to research participants, to patients, or to society. But as our field moves forward we must remember Jacob Bronowski's admonition: "No science is immune to the infection of politics and the corruption of power."

Ethical Issues for Genetic Testing

To compute the costs of health and life insurance, actuaries take into account many factors known to predict disease and death. For example, most insurance companies charge lower premiums for nonsmokers than for smokers. Their rationale is straightforward: because, on average, smokers will incur greater health care costs and will die at a younger age, the company pays out more benefits to smokers and their survivors than they do to nonsmokers and their survivors. Insurance executives reason that these increased costs should be borne by the smokers themselves. After all, why should nonsmokers pay higher insurance premiums to cover costs incurred by someone else's choice to smoke?

Few people argue with this line of reasoning. But does a parallel argument justify the use of genetic testing in the assignment of insurance premiums? Theoretically, a future actuary could have access to the genetic profiles of people who apply for insurance. If a particular profile shows an individual to have an untreatable, fatal disease (e.g., Huntington disease) or a chronic, disabling condition (e.g., schizophrenia), should that person pay higher insurance premiums? Should the insurance company have the right to exclude the affected individual from coverage?

These potential uses of genetic data by insurance companies have already affected researchers, patients, and genetic counselors. Researchers must face a very specific ethical question. Because they collect DNA from research participants, it is possible that, despite all their efforts to maintain confidentiality, the genetic data from the project might fall into the hands of an insurance company and lead to loss of insurance. To deal with this problem, researchers must inform participants about this risk when they seek the person's consent to participate.

In genetic counseling situations that use DNA tests, individual patients and family members are often concerned about health and life insurance companies' access to test results. This concern is particularly relevant in situations involving untreatable disorders such as Huntington and Alzheimer disease. At medical genetics clinics, at-risk individuals often pay for genetic testing on their own, for they fear future denial of insurance on the basis of test results. These fears are often justifiable. Thus, counselors should advise consultands to review their health, disability, and life insurance policies *prior* to genetic testing. They should also routinely discuss with them the potential implications that results might have on their future insurability. Patients should be informed that genetic testing results are part of their medical records, to which insurance companies often have access.

In the future, when genes for psychiatric disorders are known, these issues will become widespread. Psychiatric disorders are relatively common (compared, for example, with Huntington disease) and many are associated with high and chronic treatment costs. Thus, insurance companies may require presymptomatic genetic testing of common mental disorders to screen for high-risk individuals.

Like insurance companies, employers may desire to know their employees' risks for heritable diseases. Because potential employees at risk for illness may eventually be less productive and may increase a company's health care costs, some employers might discriminate on the bases of presymptomatic genetic information. Some argue that this is unjustifiable, especially for late-onset disorders that may not develop until late in life. Others reply that for occupations that involve the safety of the general public (e.g., commercial airline pilots, physicians), test results of disorders that can impair an individual's judgment and job performance should be disclosed to employers.

> **Key Point:** As tests for genetic diseases are becoming routinely available, society must be wary of the potential misuse of test data by insurance companies, employers, and others. Who should have access to your genetic information and how should it be used?

Due to the potential misuse of presymptomatic genetic testing, several guidelines have emerged for genetic counselors. First, before genetic testing begins, the individual being tested should undergo pretest counseling to learn about the ramifications of testing. The individual should also consent to the testing procedure though a process that documents his or her full understanding of the risks and benefits of receiving genetic information. The fact that a person has sought genetic testing along with the test results must be strictly confidential, but consultands must be informed of any legal limits to that confidentiality in conformance with local legislation.

Unlike most other laboratory tests, genetic test information not only affects the individual being tested but also could have an impact on other family members. Unintentionally, test results about one family member could reveal the risks of another family member. For example, finding out that a child has a gene may implicate the parent with the same mutation. Thus, testing children who do not have clinical manifestations is considered inappropriate, even if requested by parents or other authorities such as adoption agencies.

The implications of the Human Genome Project have not escaped the attention of legislators. In the United States, several states have already enacted genetic privacy laws. Although differing in detail from state to state, these laws place limits on the use of genetic data by insurance companies.

Attempts to study or legislate genetic privacy have raised several questions:

1. How should genetic privacy laws define a genetic test?
2. Should genetic test data be treated like other types of medical information?
3. Who owns the DNA samples collected from patients and research subjects?
4. Who should benefit from the commercial use of that information?

Although genetic tests are fairly well defined, there has not been complete agreement among jurisdictions as to some details of the definition. For example, some states focus attention on tests that examine DNA, RNA, or the chromosomes, whereas others employ much broader definitions, including tests of proteins encoded by a gene. Genetic privacy laws also vary in the degree to which they exclude certain standard medical tests from their reach.

The idea that genetic information should be treated differently from other clinical data has been hotly debated. Is a genetic test for the Huntington disease gene really any different from tests for high blood pressure or elevated cholesterol? One obvious difference is that the test for Huntington disease can predict with 100 percent accuracy whether patients will or will not suffer an early death. In contrast, tests for high

blood pressure and cholesterol tell patients that they are at risk for
heart disease, which is a preventable and treatable condition. In many
ways the test for the Huntington disease gene is more similar to the test
for the HIV virus. Because nearly all HIV-positive cases develop AIDS,
and because AIDS will eventually lead to death, HIV status, like Huntington disease status, predicts early death. HIV test results have been
afforded special protections under the law. Shouldn't the same be true
of Huntington disease gene status?

Although sound, the above argument begs the question: Why
should either Huntington disease gene status or HIV status be pro-
tected by the law? The answer lies in discrimination, the process
whereby we humans make distinctions among ourselves based on many
phenotypes: race, ethnicity, gender, religion, sexual orientation, social
class, physical disabilities, intelligence, physical strength, attractiveness,
and so forth. Indeed, humans have shown a remarkably flexible ability
to classify each other and to guide our behavior based on the stereo-
types that emerge from such classifications.

There are many horrible consequences of discrimination. Past
atrocities have been well preserved by historians. Current examples are
easy to find within the pages of any serious newspaper. In contrast, the
benefits of discrimination are nil. Given that so much trouble has been
caused by our easy access to many of each other's phenotypes, it makes
little sense to compound problems by allowing access to each other's
genotypes.

In 1997, the U.S. Congress approved the Health Insurance Portability and Accountability Act of 1997 (HIPAA), which provides additional protection to people who seek genetic testing. HIPAA limits the
ability of group health insurers to deny coverage based on "preexisting
conditions." Under the law, these insurance plans may deny insurance
based on a preexisting condition only when medical advice, diagnosis,
care, or treatment was recommended or received within the six-month
period before enrollment. Most unexpressed genetic conditions would
not meet this insurance exclusion requirement.

Moreover, HIPAA explicitly protects people seeking presymptomatic genetic testing. It does so by forbidding group plans from denying insurance based on genetic information when the person has not
been diagnosed with the genetic condition. This creates an important
distinction. Someday it may be possible to undergo genetic testing for
depression. Doctors may recommend preventive treatments to people
with depression genes but HIPAA would stop an insurance company
from using the recommendation as evidence of a preexisting condition. Thus, HIPAA greatly reduces the risk of genetic discrimination by
health insurance companies.

> **Key Point:** Current trends in legislation protect peo-
> ple seeking presymptomatic genetic testing from be-
> ing denied health insurance based on the results of
> their tests.

Lawmakers must also grapple with the question of who owns genetic material extracted from a specific individual. Several years ago,
scientists in California extracted unique cells from a male patient.
Without telling the patient, they used his cells to create a pharmaceutical product, the sales of which enriched the investigators and their university, but not the patient. When the patient learned about this profit-
making enterprise, he sued the investigators, claiming that the cells
were his property and that he should receive the financial benefit from
their unique properties. A California court eventually ruled that the patient did not have property rights to the cells but also ruled that the investigators had violated the patient's rights by not obtaining his
consent for participation in the research.

In the wake of the California court's ruling, other states moved to
shore up the biologic property rights of humans. In 1996, lawmakers in
New Jersey approved a law that would have dramatically expanded the
rights of individuals to retain property rights to any biologic material
they provided to researchers. The law had been opposed by scientists
and pharmaceutical companies who predicted that it would discourage
research and innovation by creating many practical difficulties. They
argued that to keep track of all individuals who had donated material
for research would be difficult enough, but to sort out who should and
who should not receive subsequent compensation would be intracta-
ble. In the end, the proposed law was vetoed by New Jersey's governor.
However, another bill was passed that required researchers to obtain
informed consent for the use of biologic materials in a manner that
would clarify to participants that, although the results could lead to a
commercially valuable product, participants would receive no financial
benefit from their participation.

Some people are troubled about the legal trend toward denying research participants rights to their biologic products. After all, your
DNA not only comes from you, it is the biologic blueprint for your
body. Why should someone else own that blueprint? The answer lies in
the concepts of intellectual and scientific freedom. If the scientists
working with DNA and other biologic samples do not have the right to
use them as they please, they will be constrained, research will not proceed, and discoveries that would be beneficial to us all will not be
made. Likewise, if individuals and companies lose the financial benefits

of their discoveries, their incentive for achieving new breakthroughs would be diminished.

You can expect the ethical and legal debates about genetic testing to continue. Indeed, they are likely to intensify if and when scientists develop the capability to predict behavioral and psychologic traits with accuracy. Then society must decide if genetic data about these traits should be given to prospective parents. Imagine that some entrepreneur decides to offer genetic counseling services to tell parents the likely intelligence and personality of their unborn child. If this sounds like fantasy, recall that the first report of animal cloning was quickly followed by a Chicago physicist's announcement that he would try to clone a human being.

Likewise, a future entrepreneur might try to sell parents on the idea that they should learn about the behavioral and psychologic traits of their unborn children. He or she might argue that future parents should be prepared to deal with the personal strengths and weaknesses of their children. Knowing that a child has genes for shyness would allow parents to plan an environment that encourages sociability. Learning that a child will be dull-witted would give parents a head start toward enriching their child's learning environment. Yet, as well intentioned as these ideas may sound, they ignore a crucial fact: having never dealt with this type of genetic data in the past, society will have no idea about the ramifications of providing it to parents.

Indeed, there are many questions that scientists, clinicians, ethicists, and legislators must consider before "genetic profiles" are given to prospective parents. What type of genetic counseling should proceed the provision of such information? Should high-achieving parents be allowed to terminate pregnancies based on the behavioral or psychologic traits of the fetus? Is it ethical to choose abortion because the fetus will "only" be of average intelligence or is likely to be an introvert?

Society must also consider if such behavioral genetic data should even be provided to prospective parents. Assuming these data could be used for good, do they also hold the potential for harm? What if two parents disagree on the desirability of a behavioral trait? Will that disrupt marriages and other family relationships? As a society becomes habituated to the idea of easy access to genetic profiles, will its members adopt a genetic fatalism that discourages attempts to improve the human lot by modifying the environment?

Although there are no easy answers to these questions, the ELSI program has established the intellectual framework needed to search for their answers. As that search proceeds, society will benefit from a cautious approach to the use of genetic data about behavioral and psychologic traits. The study of these traits may bring many medical and scientific gifts to society, but one of these may well be a Pandora's box.

Informed Consent:
The Cornerstone of Ethical Research and Practice

The guiding principle assuring the ethics of all research is the idea of informed consent. Consultands choosing genetic testing for clinical reasons should be thoroughly informed about the risks and benefits of procedures and should always have the option of terminating the counseling process. Likewise, research participants must be informed about the risks and benefits of research protocols. They must be told not only that they have the right to decline participation, but also that declining to participate will not affect their access to clinical services.

> **Key Point:** Genetic data should not be collected for either clinical or research purposes without the written informed consent of the person from whom the data are being collected.

Any informed consent process should describe the nature of the procedures, whether they are experimental or well studied, and how much time they will require. The form should use simple language to tell participants about any known risks, regardless of how improbable they may be. The risks may be physical, psychological, social, or financial. For studies involving the treatment of disease, the form must enumerate alternative procedures and their known benefits.

Consent forms should routinely describe the confidentiality of the data to be collected and, even though confidentiality may be assured by the procedures, acknowledge the adverse outcomes that would result from unforeseen violations of confidentiality. Where there are risks for injuries, the consent process should describe how such injuries would be compensated.

Consent forms must identify a person who can be contacted in case there are questions about the procedures or their results. In all cases the form must indicate that participation is voluntary, that the participant may withdraw at any time, and that there will be no loss of benefits due to withdrawal. If biologic samples are collected, the use of these samples both immediately and in the future, whether for research or for commercial purposes, must be described.

Ethical Issues for Gene Therapy

Even if they obtain our informed consent, should researchers or physicians be permitted to modify our genetic blueprint through gene therapy? The argument in favor of gene therapy is straightforward.

Physicians and other health care professionals seek to save lives and reduce distress and disability. If the modification of genes will save someone from a dreadful disease, it would seem that physicians would be obligated to provide gene therapy, even if that means tinkering with the patient's genetic code. In this view, gene therapy is simply another, albeit highly sophisticated, medical procedure. Why deny its benefits to those in need?

This line of reasoning has been generally accepted, but only in reference to the gene therapy of cells not involved in reproduction. Therapy involving somatic cells, such as bone marrow or lung tissue, will change the genetic code of these particular cells but these changes will not be transmitted to future generations. In contrast, the gene therapy of egg and sperm, the germline cells of reproduction, *will* have repercussions for future generations. Thus, germline gene therapy has been more hotly debated.

Germline gene therapy has one key advantage: it constitutes a permanent intergenerational cure. For example, imagine that gene therapy will someday be possible for Huntington disease. Should physicians only treat the somatic genes of the Huntington disease gene carrier who has not yet become ill? In that case they would prevent disease in those individuals but not in their offspring. By also treating the germline, physicians might conceivably eradicate this terrible disease. Moreover, it would save future generations from the expense, discomfort, and risk of somatic cell therapies.

Another reason not to outlaw germline therapy is that we know so little about the potential successes of somatic cell gene therapy. For example, it is conceivable that, for some diseases, scientists might develop a germline therapy but have difficulty developing a somatic cell therapy for the same disease. Shouldn't germline therapy be allowed in such cases? Finally, by outlawing germline therapy, we would stop attempts to research these techniques. By blocking this line of scientific thought, we may lose the knowledge and technologies that would otherwise have emerged.

Although germline therapy holds the potential for eradicating some genetic diseases, are there any risks associated with permanently modifying our gene pool? The only honest answer must be an admission of ignorance. We simply do not know. It is, however, easy to imagine adverse outcomes. For example, a fertile mind could generate many science fiction scenarios whereby gene therapy gone awry creates generations of madmen or monsters that wreak havoc on the earth.

Although such concerns are not realistic, a sober look at germline therapy forces us to acknowledge other possibilities. If such therapy is developed, how widely will it be applied? Even if the germline gene therapy of Huntington disease was deemed acceptable, where would we draw the line? Would germline therapy be used to treat behavioral, psychological, or emotional problems? Contemplate this example. Some researchers are currently searching for intelligence genes. When these genes are discovered will potential parents seek to modify their reproductive cells to increase the intelligence of their children? If gene therapy is expensive and only available to wealthy people, do we run the risk of creating a new class division, separating the world into the genetic haves and have-nots? Would this create a superintelligent minority that could use its endowments to maintain the superiority of its class?

There is another problem with the germline therapy of behavioral traits which, although speculative, cannot be ignored. For many years, psychiatric geneticists have been puzzled by the fact that the prevalence of some psychiatric disorders has not decreased over time despite the fact that the disorder impairs the patient's ability to reproduce. The best example is schizophrenia, which usually onsets prior to the age of reproduction and makes it difficult for those affected to develop relationships that would lead to children. In fact, the majority of schizophrenic patients do not have children. Given these facts, schizophrenia genes should be eliminated from the gene pool and the prevalence of the disorder should have diminished with time. Why has this not happened?

One possibility is that schizophrenia genes in small doses may confer survival advantages that increase the probability of reproduction. For example, maybe one or more of these genes leads to increased intelligence, enhanced creativity, gregariousness, or attractiveness. Any of these traits might have enough of an adaptive advantage to help maintain schizophrenia genes in the gene pool.

A clear medical example of this phenomenon is sickle cell anemia, a recessive genetic disorder. If you carry two copies of the mutant gene you will suffer a painful and early death. But if you carry only one copy of the mutant gene, you will not develop sickle cell disease and the mutant gene will protect you from malaria. Thus, carrying two sickle cell genes confers a reproductive disadvantage but carrying only one confers an advantage. The trade-off between the costs and benefits of the sickle cell gene means that it will not be forced out of the gene pool by the pressures of evolution.

For psychiatric disorders, the balancing of costs and benefits is not as clear. We have no proof that small doses of mental illness genes are adaptive, but theoretical considerations favor this idea. For instance, genes for panic disorder cause distress and disability and may thereby interfere with relationships and reproduction. But in low doses, genes for panic disorder might provide an appropriate level of fear and behavioral inhibition. Compared with people having no panic genes, those with low doses may be more likely to avoid dangerous situations, thereby increasing their chances of survival and reproduction.

These considerations suggest that the germline therapy of psychiatric conditions and behavioral traits could reduce the frequency of genes that, in most cases, are valuable to our species. Society may need to tolerate behavioral and social deviance and treat its adverse outcomes rather than eliminate its genetic source. Although speculative, this line of reasoning argues against germline therapy and in doing so reveals another flaw in the intellectual foundation of the eugenics movement.

Germline gene therapy raises new problems for the process of informed consent. We can imagine an informed consent procedure whereby people agree to permanent changes in their genes, but we cannot have an informed consent process for the future generation of people who will inherit a modified set of genes. Moreover, some proposals for germline gene therapy work directly on embryos, who cannot give informed consent for research participation. When we begin to question whether embryos or future generations have rights to informed consent, we are probing the very essence of what it means to be human and when human life actually begins. Because these questions have moral, political, and religious implications, their answers will likely be the subject of heated debate for many years.

Glossary

Adenine: One of four chemical bases that make up DNA. It pairs with thymine.

Affected relative pair method: The statistical analysis of pairs of affected relatives to find DNA markers linked to a disease gene. Can be used without knowing a disorder's mode of inheritance.

Affected sib-pair method: The most common form of the affected relative pair method.

Alleles: Alternative variants of a gene. Each individual has two alleles at each genetic location, one inherited from the mother and one from the father.

Amino acids: The 20 molecules that make up proteins. Genes define the sequence of amino acids required to build each protein.

Amniocentesis: A prenatal diagnostic method using cells in the amniotic fluid to examine fetal chromosomes.

Aneuploidy: Having too many or too few copies of a chromosome.

Association studies: A method that finds genes using patients and ethnically matched controls or triads made up of patients and their parents.

Autoradiography: The use of X-ray film to visualize radioactively labeled molecules for assaying the length and number of DNA fragments separated by gel electrophoresis.

Autosomal chromosome, or autosome: A chromosome having nothing to do with sex determination and development of secondary sexual characteristics. There are 22 sets of autosomes in humans. *Compare with* Sex chromosomes.

Bands: The parts of a chromosome distinguished from one another on the basis of staining.

Base: The chemical units that, in combination with other molecules, form nucleotides, the building blocks of DNA. DNA's four bases are adenine (A), thymine (T), guanine (G), and cytosine (C).

Base-pair (bp): Pairs of bases that bond to one another. Adenine bonds to thymine, guanine to cytosine. A strand of DNA consists of a sequence of these pairs. The sequence of pairs determines the function of the DNA. The number of base-pairs is often used as a measure of the length of a DNA segment.

Biotechnology: The set of biologic technologies used to create commercial products from basic research in molecular biology.

bp: Abbreviation for base-pair.

Candidate gene: A gene whose biologic function suggests that it might cause a specific disease.

Carrier: A person who carries one copy of a mutant gene but who is clinically unaffected due to the presence of one normal gene.

Carrier testing: Genetic testing that seeks to identify carriers.

Centimorgan (cM): A measure of the distance between loci on chromosomes. Two genetic loci are 1 cM apart if their probability of recombination is 1 percent. In humans, 1 cM is approximately 1 million base-pairs.

Chemical base: *See* Base.

Chorionic villus sampling: A prenatal diagnostic procedure that takes a DNA sample from the human embryo.

Chromosome: In cells, these self-replicating threadlike strands of DNA contain genes in a linear array.

Clone: Genetically engineered copies of DNA sequences, genes, cells, or organisms derived from a single ancestor.

Cloning: The procedure of making genetically identical copies of DNA sequences, genes, cells, or organisms.

cM: Abbreviation for centimorgan.

Complex trait: Any feature of an organism that has a genetic component that cannot be attributed to a single gene.

Consanguinity: The existence of a genetic relationship. Two people are consanguineous if they have at least one common ancestor in the preceding few generations.

Conservative change: A gene mutation leading to an amino acid change that does not significantly change the function of the protein.

Conserved sequence: A sequence of DNA that has not changed throughout evolution. Conserved sequences will be identical or very similar in humans and other animals.

CpG islands: Regions of DNA containing multiple repeats of the bases cytosine and guanine.

Crossing over: The exchange of genes between paired chromosomes during the formation of sperm and egg cells. Also known as recombination.

Cytogenetics: The study of the number and structure of chromosomes.

Cytosine: One of the four chemical bases that make up DNA. It pairs with guanine.

Deletion: A type of mutation in which a break in DNA causes the loss of a piece of a chromosome.

Deletion mapping: A laboratory method that uses overlapping deletions to find the location of an unknown gene.

Dinucleotide repeat: A DNA marker made up of a repeated sequence of two bases (e.g., CACACA ...). Because the number of repeats is highly variable between individuals, these markers are very useful in linkage analysis.

Diploid: Having the full set of paired chromosomes, one from each parent. Most animal cells except the gametes have a diploid set of chromosomes. The diploid human genome has 46 chromosomes.

DNA (deoxyribonucleic acid): A double-stranded molecule made up of four chemical bases: adenine (A), guanine (G), cytosine (C), and thymine (T). Genes are sequences of base-pairs within the DNA molecule.

DNA fingerprinting: A method that determines if a sample of DNA came from a specific individual.

DNA marker: A signpost at a chromosomal locus at which laboratory procedures can differentiate individuals on the composition of DNA at that location.

DNA repair genes: Genes that allow cells to fix DNA mutations. Also called proofreader genes.

DNA sequence: The order of base-pairs in a strand of DNA.

DNA sequencing: The process of determining the order of base-pairs in a strand of DNA.

Dominant allele: The version of a gene that is expressed if either one or two copies are present. A single-gene disease is described as dominant if only one copy of the pathogenic gene is needed for the disease to occur. *Compare with* Recessive allele.

Double helix: The physical shape formed by the paired strands of DNA that make up chromosomes.

Duplication: A mutation that causes a piece of a chromosome to be replicated twice.

Electrophoresis: A laboratory method that separates larger and smaller fragments of DNA from one another. The number and sizes of the fragments are used to differentiate versions of a DNA marker.

Endonuclease: An enzyme that chops DNA into fragments.

Endophenotype: A result of disease gene action that although not clinically significant and not directly observable can be measured in the laboratory. For example, attentional impairment is believed to be an endophenotype for schizophrenia.

Enzyme: A protein that facilitates a chemical process.

Epistasis: Interaction between two or more genes.

Eugenics: An ideology that believes that society can be improved by discouraging the breeding of people believed to carry undesirable genes.

Exons: Sequences of base-pairs within a gene that provide the blueprint for building a specific protein. *Compare with* Introns.

Expressivity: The extent to which a given phenotype is manifested in an individual. Many diseases have variable expressivity: some patients are severely affected, others have only mild symptoms.

FISH (fluorescence *in situ* hybridization): A laboratory method that uses fluorescent tags to identify deletion mutations.

Gametes: The reproductive cells (egg and sperm). Also called germ cells.

Gene: The unit of inheritance defined by the sequence of base-pairs in its DNA molecule. Genes contain all the information needed to create a specific biologic product.

Gene family: A group of genes that make similar products.

Gene map: The sequence of DNA markers and genes on chromosomes and the distances between them as inferred from experiments. Also known as genetic linkage map or linkage map.

Gene mapping: The process whereby scientists determine the relative positions and distances of DNA markers and genes on a chromosome. Also known as genetic linkage mapping or linkage mapping.

Gene product: The protein constructed by a gene.

Gene testing: The examination of DNA for the purpose of determining if a person is predisposed to a genetic disease.

Gene therapy: The insertion of a correctly functioning gene into cells containing malfunctioning versions of the gene.

Genetic counseling: The process whereby clinical professionals communicate recurrence risks for genetic diseases to individuals, couples, or families.

Genetic engineering technologies: Laboratory methods used to create new sequences of DNA or to modify existing sequences. These sequences may then be inserted in living cells to study or capitalize on their biologic activity.

Genetic heterogeneity: The existence of more than one genetic cause for a single disease.

Genetic linkage map: The sequence of DNA markers and genes on chromosomes and the distances between them as inferred from experiments. Also known as gene map or linkage map.

Genetic linkage mapping: The process whereby scientists determine the relative positions and distances of DNA markers and genes on a chromosome. Also known as gene mapping or linkage mapping.

Genetic screening: A clinical program that tests groups of people to find those at risk for specific genetic diseases.

Genome: The complete DNA content of a cell.

Genotype: When used in reference to an individual, the pair of genes that a person has at a specified chromosomal location. When used in reference to a disease, the gene or set of genes required for disease expression.

Germ cells: The reproductive cells (egg and sperm). Also called gametes.

Germline mutation: A mutation that affects egg or sperm and is therefore transmitted to offspring. Also known as hereditary mutation. *Compare with* Somatic mutation.

Goodness of fit: Used to describe the ability of a statistical model to describe data. We say a model has a "good fit" if it accurately predicts the observed data.

Guanine: One of the four chemical bases that make up DNA. It pairs with cytosine.

Haploid: Having only one copy of each chromosome. In animals, most cells are diploid (they have two copies). The gametes are haploid.

Hereditary mutation: A mutation that affects egg or sperm and is therefore transmitted to offspring. Also known as germline mutation. *Compare with* somatic mutation.

Heterozygote: An individual is heterozygous if two alleles at a particular locus are different.

Homologies: Similarities in DNA among different species. *See* Conserved sequence.

Homologous chromosomes: A pair of chromosomes containing the same sequence of genes. One member of the pair came from the mother, the other from the father. When egg and sperm are created, members of a pair cross over and exchange genetic information. Only one of the two resulting chromosomes is transmitted to offspring.

Homozygote: An individual is homozygous if two alleles at a given locus are the same.

Human Genome Project: A project led by the National Institutes of Health and the Department of Energy that seeks to completely sequence the human genome.

Hybridization: The process of joining two complementary strands of DNA to form a double-stranded molecule.

Hybridize: The process whereby a strand of DNA "sticks to" or identifies its complementary strand in a mixture of DNA molecules.

Identical by descent: Two alleles in two people are identical by descent if they are both copies of a gene transmitted from the same ancestor. *Compare with* Identical by state.

Identical by state: Two alleles in two people are identical by state if they are made up of the same DNA sequence regardless of whether they were inherited from the same ancestor. *Compare with* Identical by descent.

Imprinting: A biologic process that modifies genes in a manner that is dependent on the sex of the parent. Thus, the effects of imprinted genes depend on which parent transmitted them.

In vitro: A biologic or chemical process that occurs in the laboratory outside of a living organism.

Incomplete penetrance: This term describes disease genes that only sometimes lead to disease.

Informativeness: A characteristic describing how useful DNA markers are for genetic linkage studies. Informativeness increase with the number of different versions of the marker that occur in the family. *See also* Polymorphism information content

Insertion: A mutation caused by the insertion of additional DNA into a chromosome.

Introns: Sequences of base-pairs within a gene that interrupt the sequences that provide the blueprint for building a specific protein. *Compare with* Exons.

Inversion: A mutation caused when two breaks in a chromosome excise a piece of DNA and that DNA is then reinserted into the chromosome in reverse order.

Karyotype: A photograph of the chromosomes showing the number, size, and shape of each chromosome.

Karyotyping: A laboratory procedure that creates karyotypes with the goal of finding structural and numeric abnormalities in chromosomes.

kb: Abbreviation for kilobase.

Kilobase (kb): 1,000 base-pairs of DNA sequence.

Knockout: Inactivation of a gene by laboratory procedures.

Landmark: In cytogenetics, a term describing consistent structural features that identify individual chromosomes.

Liability: The unobservable genetic predisposition to developing a disease.

Likelihood: The result of a computation that indexes the probability of having observed a set of data if a specific model of genetic transmission were true.

Linkage: The nearness of two or more genes or markers on a chromosome; as the genetic distance decreases, the probability that they will be inherited together increases.

Linkage analysis: A statistical gene-hunting method that traces patterns of heredity based on the tendency of two alleles at different loci on the same chromosome to be inherited together.

Linkage disequilibrium: Two genes or DNA markers are said to be in linkage disequilibrium if people having one version of one gene (or marker) are highly likely to have a specific version of the other gene (or marker). This usually occurs when genes are so close together that they have not been completely reshuffled by recombination.

Linkage map: The sequence of DNA markers and genes on chromosomes and the distances between them as inferred from experiments. Also known as genetic linkage map or gene map.

Linkage mapping: The process whereby scientists determine the relative positions and distances of DNA markers and genes on a chromosome. Also known as genetic linkage mapping or gene mapping.

Loci: Plural of Locus.

Locus: The location of a gene or marker on a chromosome.

Lod score: Literally refers to the log of an odds ratio, a statistic that is used to quantify the degree to which data support or reject the hypothesis of genetic linkage.

Mapping: *See* Gene mapping.

Marker: A physical location on a chromosome that can be detected with laboratory procedures. *See* DNA marker.

Mb: Abbreviation for megabase.

Megabase (Mb): A unit of length for DNA equal to 1 million base-pairs and equal to about 1 cM.

Meiosis: In humans, the biological process that creates sperm and egg cells.

Mendelian inheritance: The transmission from parent to offspring of traits or diseases in a dominant or recessive fashion as first reported by Gregor Mendel. The term is synonymous with single gene locus.

Microsatellites: A type of genetic marker. Also known as tandem dinucleotide repeats.

Missense mutation: A change in the base sequence of a gene that garbles the genetic code and prevents the synthesis of a protein.

Mitochondria: That part of a cell that produces energy.

Mitochondrial DNA: A circular piece of DNA found in the mitochondria.

Mitochondrial inheritance: Transmission of a trait or disease through genes contained in mitochondrial DNA.

Mode of transmission: The mechanism whereby traits or diseases are transmitted from parents to children.

Multifactorial polygenic inheritance: A mode of transmission whereby a large, unspecified number of genes and environmental factors combine in an additive fashion to cause a disease or trait. *Compare with* Oligogenic inheritance; Polygenic disorders; Single major gene.

Mutation: A permanent change in the DNA molecule that modifes the number, arrangement, or base-pair sequence of one or more genes.

Newborn screening: The examination of newborn infants to detect genetic abnormalities.

Nitrogenous base: *See* Base.

Nonsense mutation: A mutation that results in the gene making a truncated and therefore useless protein product.

Nucleotide: A base plus the phosphate and sugar molecules needed to form DNA.

Nucleus: That part of the cell that contains the chromosomes.

Oligogenic inheritance: A mode of transmission whereby several genes act additively or interactively to produce a disease or trait. Oligogenic transmission, which involves a relatively small set of genes, differs from polygenic and multifactorial transmission, which require the combined actions of many genes. *Compare with* Single major gene.

P arm: The short arm of a chromosome. *Compare with* Q arm.

Path analysis: A statistical method that partitions genetic and environmental contributions to traits in a sample of families.

Path coefficients: A measure of the strength of the association between two variables.

PCR: Abbreviation for polymerase chain reaction.

Pedigree: A graphic representation of a family of study using standard symbols.

Penetrance: The probability that a person carrying a disease-predisposing gene will develop that disease.

Phage: A virus that attacks a bacterial cell.

Phenocopy: An individual who exhibits a trait without carrying the gene that causes the trait (i.e., a nongenetic copy of a phenotype that can also be caused by genes).

Phenotype: An observable trait or disease.

Physical map: A map of a chromosome or chromosome segment in which the distance between markers is an actual physical measurement, such as the number of base-pairs. For humans, the lowest resolution physical map is the banding patterns on the 24 different chromosomes; the highest resolution map would be the complete base-pair sequence of the chromosomes.

Pleiotropy: The existence of more than one phenotype being caused by a gene or set of genes.

Polygenic disorders: Genetic disorders resulting from the additive action of a large number of genes. The term "multifactorial polygenic" is usually used when many environmental factors also add to the predisposition to disease. *Compare with* Oligogenic inheritance; Single major gene.

Polymerase chain reaction (PCR): A technique for copying strands of DNA simultaneously for a series of cycles to create many copies of the strand.

Polymorphism: A gene or DNA marker showing differences in its sequence among individuals. If more than one variant occurs in more than 1 percent of a population, the gene or marker is considered polymorphic.

Polymorphism information content (PIC): A measure describing how useful DNA markers are for genetic linkage studies. PIC, or informativeness, increase with the number of different versions of the marker that occur in the family.

Positional cloning: The identification of a gene without knowing its gene product, using linkage analysis and laboratory methods. Also known as reverse genetics.

Predictive genetic tests: Tests that identify gene abnormalities that make a person susceptible to specific diseases.

Prenatal diagnosis: The testing of fetal cells for biochemical or genetic defects.

Presymptomatic diagnosis: Diagnosis of a genetic disease before the appearance of its symptoms.

Probability: The frequency of an outcome relative to all other possible outcomes, expressed as a decimal number between 0 and 1 or a percentage between zero percent and 100 percent. In both cases, higher numbers correspond to more probable events.

Proband: The member or members of a family who are selected for a research study.

Promoter: That part of a gene that controls the initiation of protein production.

Proofreader genes: Genes that allow cells to fix DNA mutations. Also called DNA repair genes.

Protein: A large molecule essential to the structure, function, and regulation of the body. The structure and function of a protein are determined by its sequence of amino acids. The sequence of amino acids is coded in the sequence of the base-pairs in the gene that creates the protein.

Purine: A nitrogen-containing, single-ring, basic compound that occurs in nucleic acids. The purines in DNA and RNA are adenine and guanine.

Q arm: The long arm of a chromosome. *Compare with* P arm.

Quantitative trait: A trait that is continuous (i.e., follows the normal bell-shape distribution in the general population), such as height and intelligence.

Recessive allele: The version of a gene that is expressed only if two copies are present. A single-gene disease is described as recessive if two copies of the pathogenic gene are needed for the disease to occur. *Compare with* Dominant allele.

Recombinant DNA molecules: Novel or modified sequences of DNA created in the laboratory.

Recombinant DNA technologies: Laboratory methods used to create novel or modified sequences of DNA. These sequences may then be inserted in living cells to study or capitalize on their biological activity.

Recombination: The exchange of genes between paired chromosomes during the formation of sperm and egg cells. This process leads to offspring that have a combination of genes different from that of either parent. Also known as crossing over.

Recombination fraction: The probability that two alleles on the same chromosome will end up on different chromosomes during the creation of egg and sperm. It is expressed as a number between 0 and .5; the lower the recombination fraction, the closer two genes are to one another.

Regulatory regions: A DNA sequence that controls the timing or amount of gene expression.

Repeat sequences: A DNA sequence that is repeated several times. These sequences make useful markers because individuals will differ in the number of times the sequence is repeated at a specific locus. Also called tandem repeat sequences.

Replication: The process of making an identical new pair of chromosomes by using one strand of its DNA as the template for making the opposite strand.

Reproductive cells: Egg and sperm cells. Also called gametes or germ cells.

Resolution: Degree of detail on a physical map of DNA.

Restriction enzymes: Enzymes that can cut strands of DNA at specific base sequences.

Restriction fragment length polymorphism (RFLP): When a restriction enzyme is used to digest DNA, chromosomal regions are cut into specific fragments. Some of these fragment lengths are variable between individuals. Loci where this is the case are RFLPs; they provide convenient DNA markers for linkage analysis.

Reverse genetics: The identification of a gene without knowing its gene product, using linkage analysis and laboratory methods. Also known as positional cloning.

RFLP: Acronym for restriction fragment length polymorphism.

Segregation: The separation of paired chromosomes at the time of egg or sperm formation.

Segregation analysis: A mathematical modeling procedure applied to family study data that determines the mode of transmission of a disease or trait.

Sequence: The order of base-pairs in a strand of DNA.

Sequence tagged site (STS): A short (less than 500 base-pair) DNA sequence, having a known location and base sequence, that occurs once in the human genome.

Sequencing: The process of determining the order of base-pairs in a strand of DNA.

Sex chromosomes: The chromosomes that determine the sex of an organism. Human females have two X chromosomes; males have one X and one Y. *Compare with* autosomal chromosome.

Single-gene disorder: Hereditary disorder caused by mutation of a single gene (e.g., Duchenne muscular dystrophy, retinoblastoma, sickle cell disease). *Compare with* Multifactorial polygenic inheritance; Oligogenic inheritance; Polygenic inheritance.

Single major gene: The presence of gene that exerts a major effect in the expression of the phenotype. *See* Mendelian inheritance.

Somatic cells: All body cells except the reproductive cells.

Somatic mutation: A mutation that affects any cell other than egg or sperm and is therefore not transmitted to offspring. *Compare with* Germline mutation and Hereditary mutation.

STS: Acronym for sequence tagged site.

Tandem repeat sequences: A DNA sequence that is repeated several times. These sequences make useful markers because people will differ in the number of times the sequence is repeated at a specific locus. Also called repeat sequences.

Telomeres: The ends of chromosomes.

Teratogen: Any environmental agent that causes birth defects.

Thymine: One of the four chemical bases that make up DNA. It pairs with adenine.

Transgenic organism: An organism into which foreign DNA has been inserted. The resulting organism will then transmit the foreign DNA to offspring. This allows scientists to study the effects of human genes and also allows them to use animals to generate human biological material. For example, the insertion of the human insulin gene into a sheep's milk production gene would create sheep that produce milk that contains insulin. The insulin can then be extracted from the milk and used to manage diabetes.

Translocation: A mutation in which a piece of a chromosome breaks off and is reattached to a different chromosome.

Transmission disequilibrium test (TDT): A statistical test that uses a sample of ill people and their parents to test for linkage disequilibrium.

Trisomy: The condition of having three copies of a chromosome or a part of a chromosome instead of the usual two copies.

VAPSE: Acronym for a DNA sequence variation affecting the protein structure or expression.

Virus: A biological entity that uses cells from other organisms to reproduce itself. Viruses consist of DNA covered by a protein coat. Although best known for their ability to cause disease, they are also used by molecular geneticists to insert DNA into cells.

X chromosome: One of the sex chromosomes. Females have two X chromosomes. Males have one X and one Y chromosome.

X-linked disease: A disease caused by a gene on the X chromosome. These diseases show characteristic, sex-specific, patterns of inheritance.

Y chromosome: One of the sex chromosomes. Males carry one Y and one X chromosome. Females have two X chromosomes.

Readings
in Psychiatric Genetics

*T*here is a huge scientific literature describing methods and findings in psychiatric genetics. The selection listed below includes textbook presentations, useful summaries, and detailed descriptions of projects we have used as illustrations of specific methods. The references to Chapter 6 include reviews of genetic studies of most psychiatric disorders. These provide recurrence risk information that will be useful for genetic counseling.

CHAPTER 1: INTRODUTION

Faraone, S. V., & Santangelo, S. (1992). Methods in genetic epidemiology. In M. Fava & J. F. Rosenbaum (Eds.), *Research designs and methods in psychiatry*. Amsterdam, The Netherlands: Elsevier.

Faraone, S. V., & Tsuang, M. T. (1995). Methods in psychiatric genetics. In M. T. Tsuang, M. Tohen, & G. E. P. Zahner (Eds.), *Textbook in psychiatric epidemiology* (pp. 81–134). New York: Wiley-Liss.

Plomin, R. (1990). *Nature and nurture: An introduction to human behavioral genetics*. Belmont, CA: Wadsworth.

Plomin, R. (1990). The role of inheritance in behavior. *Science, 248,* 183–188.

Plomin, R., Defries, J. C., & McLearn, G. E. (1990). *Behavioral genetics: A primer* (2nd ed.). New York: Freeman.

Thompson, M. W., McInnes, R. R., & Willard, H. F. (1991). *Thompson & Thompson genetics in medicine* (5th ed.). Philadelphia: Saunders.

Tsuang, M. T. (1980). *Genes and the mind: Inheritance of mental illness*. Oxford, UK: Oxford University Press.

Vogel, F., & Motulsky, A. G. (1986). *Human genetics: Problems and approaches* (2nd ed.). Berlin: Springer-Verlag.

CHAPTER 2: THE BASICS: EPIDEMIOLOGIC FOUNDATIONS OF PSYCHIATRIC GENETICS

Andreasen, N. C. (1986). The family history approach to diagnosis: How useful is it? *Archives of General Psychiatry, 43,* 421–429.

Andreasen, N. C., Endicott, J., Spitzer, R. L., & Winokur, G. (1977). The family history method using diagnostic criteria: Reliability and validity. *Archives of General Psychiatry, 34,* 1229–1235.

Faraone, S., Biederman, J., Chen, W. J., Krifcher, B., Keenan, K., Moore, C., Sprich, S., & Tsuang, M. (1992). Segregation analysis of attention deficit hyperactivity disorder: Evidence for single gene transmission. *Psychiatric Genetics, 2,* 257–275.

Gottesman, I. I., & Shields, J. (1972). *Schizophrenia and genetics: A twin study vantage point.* New York: Academic Press.

Heston, L. L. (1966). Psychiatric disorders in foster home–reared children of schizophrenic mothers. *British Journal of Psychiatry, 112,* 819–825.

Kendler, K. S., Silberg, J. L., Neale, M. C., Kessler, R. C., Heath, A. C., & Eaves, L. J. (1991). The family history method: Whose psychiatric history is measured? *American Journal of Psychiatry, 148*(11), 1501–1504.

Kety, S. S., Rosenthal, D., Wender, P. H., & Schulsinger, F. (1968). The types and prevalence of mental illness in the biological and adoptive families of adopted schizophrenics. *Journal of Psychiatric Research, 1*(Suppl.), 345–362.

Kety, S. S., Rosenthal, D., Wender, P. H., Schulsinger, F., & Jacobson, B. (1978). The biologic and adoptive families of adopted individuals who became schizophrenic: Prevalence of mental illness and other characteristics. In L. C. Wynne, R. L. Cromwell, & S. Matthysse (Eds.), *The nature of schizophrenia: New approaches to research and treatment* (pp. 25–37). New York: Wiley.

Kety, S. S., Wender, P. H., Jacobsen, B., Ingraham, L. J., Jansson, L., Faber, B., & Kinney, D. K. (1994). Mental illness in the biological and adoptive relatives of schizophrenic adoptees: Replication of the Copenhagen Study in the rest of Denmark. *Archives of General Psychiatry, 51,* 442–455.

Khoury, M. J., Beaty, T. H., & Cohen, B. H. (1993). *Fundamentals of genetic epidemiology.* New York: Oxford University Press.

Lyons, M. J., True, W. R., Eisen, S. A., Goldberg, J., Meyer, J. M., Faraone, S. V., Eaves, L. J., & Tsuang, M. T. (1995). Differential heritability of adult and juvenile antisocial traits. *Archives of General Psychiatry, 52,* 906–915.

Mendlewicz, J., & Rainer, J. D. (1977). Adoption study supporting genetic transmission in manic–depressive illness. *Nature, 268,* 327–329.

Morton, N. E. (1982). *Outline of genetic epidemiology.* Basel, Switzerland: Karger.

Onstad, S., Skre, I., Torgersen, S., & Kringlen, E. (1991). Twin concordance for DSM-III-R schizophrenia. *Acta Psychiatrica Scandinavica, 83,* 395–401.

Tsuang, M. T., & Faraone, S. V. (1990). *The genetics of mood disorders.* Baltimore: Johns Hopkins University Press.

CHAPTER 3: VARIATIONS ON A THEME:
CAUSAL AND CLINICAL HETEROGENEITY

Biederman, J., Faraone, S. V., Keenan, K., & Tsuang, M. T. (1991). Evidence of familial association between attention deficit disorder and major affective disorders. *Archives of General Psychiatry, 48,* 633–642.

Blashfield, R. K., McElroy, R. A. Jr., Pfohl, B., & Blum, N. (1994). Comorbidity and the prototype model. *Clinical Psychological Science Practice, 1,* 96–99.

Boyd, J. H., Burke, J. D., Gruenberg, E., Holzer, C. E., Rae, D. S., George, L. K., Karno, M., Stoltzman, R., McEvoy, L., & Nestadt, G. (1984). Exclusion criteria of DSM-III: A study of co-occurrence of hierarchy-free syndromes. *Archives of General Psychiatry, 41,* 983–989.

Cannon, T. D., Mednick, S. A., & Parnas, J. (1989). Genetic and perinatal determinants of structural brain deficits in schizophrenia. *Archives of General Psychiatry, 46,* 883–889.

Cannon, T. D., Mednick, S. A., Parnas, J., Schulsinger, F., Praestholm, J., & Vestergaard, A. (1993). Developmental brain abnormalities in the offspring of schizophrenic mothers: I. Contributions of genetic and perinatal factors. *Archives of General Psychiatry, 50,* 551–564.

Caron, C., & Rutter, M. (1991). Comorbidity in child psychopathology: Concepts, issues, and research strategies. *Journal of Child Psychology and Psychiatry, 32*(7), 1063–1080.

Daniel, D. G., Goldberg, T. E., Givvons, R. D., & Weinberger, D. R. (1991). Lack of a bimodal distribution of ventricular size in schizophrenia: A Gaussian mixture analysis of 1,056 cases and controls. *Biological Psychiatry, 30,* 887–903.

Eaves, L. J., Kendler, K. S., & Schulz, S. C. (1986). The familial sporadic classification: Its power for the resolution of genetic and environmental etiological factors. *Journal of Psychiatric Research, 20,* 115–130.

Faraone, S. V., & Biederman, J. (1997). Do attention deficit hyperactivity disorder and major depression share familial risk factors? *Journal of Nervous and Mental Disease, 185*(9), 533–541.

Faraone, S. V., et al. (1993). Evidence for independent transmission in families for attention deficit hyperactivity disorder (ADHD) and learning disability: Results from a family-genetic study of ADHD. *American Journal of Psychiatry, 150,* 891–895.

Faraone, S. V., Seidman, L. J., Kremen, W. S., Pepple, J. R., Lyons, M. J., & Tsuang, M. T. (1995). Neuropsychological functioning among the nonpsychotic relatives of schizophrenic patients: A diagnostic efficiency analysis. *Journal of Abnormal Psychology, 104,* 286–304.

Gottesman, I. I. (1991). *Schizophrenia genesis: The origin of madness.* New York: Freeman.

Gottesman, I. I., & Shields, J. (1982). *Schizophrenia: The epigenetic puzzle.* Cambridge, UK: Cambridge University Press.

Lewis, S. W., Reveley, A. M., Reveley, M. A., Chitkara, B., & Murray, R. M. (1987). The familial/sporadic distinction as a strategy in schizophrenia research. *British Journal of Psychiatry, 151,* 306–313.

Lilienfeld, S. O., Waldman, I. D., & Israel, A. C. (1994). A critical examination of the use of the term and concept of comorbidity in psychopathology research. *Clinical Psychological Science Practice, 1,* 71–83.

Lyons, M. J., Faraone, S. V., Kremen, W. S., & Tsuang, M. T. (1989). Familial and sporadic schizophrenia: A simulation study of statistical power. *Schizophrenia Research, 2,* 345–353.

Moldin, S. O., & Erlenmeyer-Kimling, L. (1994). Measuring liability to schizophrenia: Progress report 1994: Editor's introduction. *Schizophrenia Bulletin, 20*(1), 25–30.

Rieder, R. O., & Gershon, E. S. (1978). Genetic strategies in biological psychiatry. *Archives of General Psychiatry, 35,* 866–873.

Rosenbaum, J. F., Biederman, J., Bolduc-Murphy, E. A., Faraone, S. V., Chaloff, J., Hirshfeld, D. R., & Kagan, J. (1993). Behavioral inhibition in childhood: A risk factor for anxiety disorders. *Harvard Review of Psychiatry, 1,* 2–16.

Roy, M.-A., & Crowe, R. R. (1994). Validity of the familial and sporadic subtypes of schizophrenia. *American Journal of Psychiatry, 151*(6), 805–814.

Rutter, M. (1994). Comorbidity: Meanings and mechanisms. *Clinical Psychological Science Practice, 1,* 100–103.

Seidman, L. J., Faraone, S. V., Goldstein, J. M., Goodman, J. M., Kremen, W. S., Matsuda, G., Hoge, E. A., Kennedy, D. N., Makris, N., Caviness, V. S., & Tsuang, M. T. (1997). Reduced subcortical brain volumes in nonpsychotic siblings of schizophrenic patients: A pilot MRI study. *American Journal of Medical Genetics: Neuropsychiatric Genetics, 74,* 507–514.

Spitzer, R. L. (1994). Psychiatric "co-ocurrence"? I'll stick with "comorbidity." *Clinical Psychological Science Practice, 1,* 88–92.

Tsuang, M. T., & Faraone, S. V. (1990). *The genetics of mood disorders.* Baltimore: Johns Hopkins University Press.

Tsuang, M. T., Winokur, G., & Crowe, R. R. (1980). Morbidity risks of schizophrenia and affective disorders among first-degree relatives of patients with schizophrenia, mania, depression, and surgical conditions. *British Journal of Psychiatry, 137,* 497–504.

CHAPTER 4: MATHEMATICAL MODELS OF INHERITANCE

Eaves, L. J. (1987). Including the environment in models for genetic segregation. *Journal of Psychiatric Research, 21*(4), 639–647.

Elston, R. C. (1981). Segregation analysis. In H. Hams & K. Hirschhorn (Eds.), *Advances in human genetics* (pp. 63–120). New York: Plenum Press.

Elston, R. C., & Yelverton, K. C. (1975). General models for segregation analysis. *American Journal of Human Genetics, 27*(1), 31–45.

Khoury, M., Beaty, T., & Cohen, B. (1993). Genetic approaches to familial aggregation: II. Segregation analysis. In *Fundamentals of genetic epidemiology* (pp. 233–283). New York: Oxford University Press.

Lalouel, J. M., Rao, D. C., Morton, N. E., & Elston, R. C. (1983). A unified model for complex segregation analysis. *American Journal of Human Genetics, 35,* 816–826.

Morton, N. E., Rao, D. C., & Lalouel, J.-M. (1983). *Methods in genetic epidemiology* (Vol. 4). New York: Karger.

Neale, M. C., & Cardon, L. R. (1992). *Methodology for genetic studies of twins and families.* Dordrecht, The Netherlands: Kluwer Academic.

Reich, T., Rice, J., Cloninger, C. R., Wette, R., & James, J. W. (1979). The use of multiple thresholds and segregation analysis in analyzing the phenotypic heterogeneity of multifactorial traits. *Annals of Human Genetics, 42,* 371–389.

Thompson, E. A. (1986). *Pedigree analysis in human genetics.* Baltimore: Johns Hopkins University Press.

CHAPTER 5: MOLECULAR GENETICS AND MENTAL ILLNESS

Bassett, A. S. (1996). Chromosomal aberrations and schizophrenia. *British Journal of Psychiatry, 161,* 323–334.

Caron, M. G. (1996). Images in neuroscience. Molecular biology, II. A dopamine transporter mouse knockout. *American Journal of Psychiatry, 153,* 1515.

Crabbe, J., Belknap, J., & Buck, K. (1994). Genetic animal models of alcohol and drug abuse. Science, *264,* 1715–1723.

Crowe, R. R. (1993). Candidate genes in psychiatry: An epidemiological perspective. *American Journal of Medical Genetics: Neuropsychiatric Genetics, 48*(2), 74–77.

Gershon, E. S., & Cloninger, C. R. (1994). *Genetic approaches to mental disorders.* Washington, DC: American Psychiatric Press.

Khoury, M. J., Adams, M. J. Jr., & Flanders, W. D. (1988). An epidemiologic approach to ecogenetics. *American Journal of Human Genetics, 42,* 89–95.

Kidd, K. K. (1993). Associations of disease with genetic markers: Deja vu all over again. *American Journal of Medical Genetics, Neuropsychiatric Genetics, 48*(2), 71–73.

Lander, E., & Kruglyak, L. (1995). Genetic dissection of complex traits: Guidelines for interpreting and reporting linkage results. *Nature Genetics, 11,* 241–247.

Lander, E. S., & Schork, N. J. (1994). Genetic dissection of complex traits. *Science, 265,* 2037–2048

Majzoub, J., & Muglia, L. (1996). Knockout mice. *New England Journal of Medicine, 334,* 904–907.

McConkey, E. H. (1993). Human genetics: The molecular revolution. Boston: Jones & Bartlett.

Ott, J. (1991). *Analysis of human genetic linkage* (2nd ed.). Baltimore: Johns Hopkins University Press.

Schellenberg, G. D., Bird, T. D., Wijsman, E. M., Orr, H. T., Anderson, L., Nemens, E., White, J. A., Bonnycastle, L., Weber, J. L., Alonso, M. E., Potter, H., Heston, L. L., & Martin, G. M. (1992). Genetic linkage evidence for a familial Alzheimer's disease locus on chromosome 14. *Science, 259,* 668–671.

Sobell, J. L., Heston, L. L., & Sommer, S. S. (1993). Novel association approach for determining the genetic predisposition to schizophrenia: Case–control resource and testing of a candidate gene. *American Journal of Medical Genetics: Neuropsychiatric Genetics, 48*(1), 28–35.

Spielman, R. S., McGinnis, R. E., & Ewens, W. J. (1993). Transmission test for linkage disequilibrium: The insulin gene region and insulin-dependent diabetes mellitus (IDDM). *American Journal of Human Genetics, 52*, 506–516.

Terwilliger, J., & Ott, J. (1994). *Handbook of human genetic linkage.* Baltimore: Johns Hopkins University Press.

Thompson, M. W., McInnes, R. R., & Willard, H. F. (1991). *Thompson & Thompson genetics in medicine* (5th ed.). Philadelphia: Saunders.

Weeks, D. E., & Lange, K. (1988). The affected-pedigree-member method of linkage analysis. *American Journal of Human Genetics, 42*, 315–326.

CHAPTER 6: CLINICAL APPLICATIONS OF PSYCHIATRIC GENETICS

Begleiter, H., & Kissin, B. (1995). *The genetics of alcoholism.* Oxford, UK: Oxford University Press.

Bennett, R. (1995). The genetic family history in primary care. *Genetics Northwest, 10*, 6–10

Blacker, D. (1997). The genetics of Alzheimer's disease: Progress, possibilities, and pitfalls. *Harvard Review of Psychiatry, 5*(4), 234–237.

Brennan, P. A., & Mednick, S. A. (1993). Genetic perspectives on crime. *Acta Psychiatrica Scandinavica, 87*(Suppl. 2), 19–26.

Carey, G., & DiLalla, D. L. (1994). Personality and psychopathology: Genetic perspectives. *Journal of Abnormal Psychology, 103*, 32–43.

Crabbe, J. C., Belknap, J. K., & Buck, K. J. (1994). Genetic animal models of drug abuse. *Science, 264*, 1715–1723.

Crowe, R. R. (1991). Genetic studies of anxiety disorders. In M. T. Tsuang, K. K. Kendler, & M. J. Lyons (Eds.), *Genetic issues in psychosocial epidemiology* (pp. 175–190). New Brunswick, NJ: Rutgers University Press.

DeFries, J. C., & Alarcon, M. (1996). Genetics of specific reading disability. *Mental Retardation and Developmental Disabilities Research Reviews, 2*, 39–47.

Devor, E. J. (1990). Untying the Gordian knot: The genetics of Tourette syndrome. *Journal of Nervous and Mental Disease, 178*(11), 669–679.

Dewji, N. N., & Singer, S. J. (1996). Genetic clues to Alzheimer's disease. *Science, 271*, 159–160.

Dinwiddie, S. H., & Reich, T. (1993). Genetic and family studies in psychiatric illness and alcohol and drug dependence. *Journal of Addiction Disorders, 12*, 17–27.

Faraone, S., & Biederman, J. (1994). Genetics of attention-deficit hyperactivity disorder. *Child and Adolescent Psychiatric Clinics of North America, 3*(2), 285–302.

Farmer, A., & Owen, M. J. (1996). Genomics: The next psychiatric revolution? *British Journal of Psychiatry, 169*, 135–138.

Harris, R. A., & Crabbe, J. Jr. (1991). *An overview: The genetic basis of alcohol and drug actions.* New York: Plenum Press.

McGuffin, P., & Thapar, A. (1992). The genetics of personality disorder. *British Journal of Psychiatry, 160*, 12–23.

McHugh, P. R., & McKusick, V. (1991). *Genes, brain, and behavior.* New York: Raven Press.

Merikangas, K. R. (1990). Comorbidity of anxiety and depression: Review of family-genetic studies. In J. D. Maser & C. R. Cloninger (Eds.), *Comorbidity of mood and anxiety disorders* (pp. 331–348). Washington, DC: American Psychiatric Press.

Merikangas, K. R. (1990). The genetic epidemiology of alcoholism. *Psychological Medicine, 20,* 11–22.

Miles, D. R., & Carey, G. (1997). Genetic and environmental architecture of human aggression. *Journal of Personality and Social Psychology, 72*(1), 207–217.

Moldin, S. O. (1997). Psychiatric genetic counseling. In S. B. Guze (Ed.), *Washington University adult psychiatry* (pp. 365–381). St. Louis: Mosby.

Nigg, J. T., & Goldsmith, H. H. (1994). Genetics of personality disorders: Perspectives from personality and psychopathology research. *Psychological Bulletin, 115*(3), 346–380.

Nurnberger, J. I., & Berrettini, W. (1997). *Psychiatric genetics.* New York: Chapman & Hall.

Pauls, D. L. (1992). The genetics of obsessive compulsive disorder and Gilles de la Tourette's syndrome. *Psychiatric Clinics of North America, 15*(4), 759–775.

St. Clair, D. (1994). Genetics of Alzheimer's disease: Some molecular understanding of a diverse phenotype. *British Journal of Psychiatry, 164,* 153–156.

Todd, R. D., & Heath, A. (1996). The genetic architecture of depression and anxiety in youth. *Current Opinion in Psychiatry, 9,* 257–261.

Tsuang, M. T. (1978). Genetic counseling for psychiatric patients and their families. *American Journal of Psychiatry, 135*(12), 1465–1475.

Tsuang, M. T., & Faraone, S. V. (1990). *The genetics of mood disorders.* Baltimore: Johns Hopkins University Press.

Tsuang, M. T., & Faraone, S. V. (1994). Epidemiology and behavioral genetics of schizophrenia. In S. J. Watson (Ed.), *Biology of schizophrenia and affective disease* (pp. 163–195). New York: NY: Raven Press.

Tsuang, M. T., & Faraone, S. V. (1996). The inheritance of mood disorders. In L. L. Hall (Ed.), *Genetics and mental illness: Evolving issues for research and society* (pp. 79–222). New York: Plenum Press.

Tsuang, M. T., Faraone, S. V., & Lyons, M. J. (1993). Advances in psychiatric genetics. In J. A. Costa de Silva, C. C. Nadelson, N. C. Andreasen, & M. Sato (Eds.), *International Review of Psychiatry* (Vol. 1, pp. 395–440). Washington, DC: American Psychiatric Press.

Vandenberg, S. G., Singer, S. M., & Pauls, D. L. (1986). *Heredity of behavior disorders in adults and children.* New York: Plenum Press.

CHAPTER 7: THE FUTURE OF PSYCHIATRIC GENETICS

Ad Hoc Committee on Genetic Testing/Insurance Issues. (1995). Background statement: Genetic testing and insurance. *American Journal of Human Genetics, 56,* 327–331.

American Society of Human Genetics Board of Directors and the American College of Medical Genetics Board of Directors. (1995). Points to consider: Ethical, legal, and psychosocial implications of genetic testing in children and adolescents. *American Journal of Human Genetics, 57,* 1234–1241.

Bennett, R. L., Bird, T. D., & Teri, L. (1993). Offering predictive testing for Huntington's disease in a medical genetics clinic. *Journal of Genetic Counseling, 2,* 123–137.

Bird, T. D., & Bennett, R. L. (1995). Why do DNA testing? Practical and ethical implications of new neurogenetic tests. *Annals of Neurology, 38,* 141–146.

Blau, H. M., & Springer, M. L. (1993). Molecular medicine: Gene therapy—A novel form of drug delivery. *New England Journal of Medicine, 333,* 1204–1207.

Crystal, R. G. (1995). Transfer of genes to humans: Early lessons and obstacles to success. *Science, 20,* 404–410.

Ferguson, M. (1998). The process of genetic testing for nurses and their patients. In D. H. Lea, J. F. Jenkins, & C. A. Francomano (Eds.), *Genetics in clinical practice* (pp. 145–175). Sudbury, MA: Jones & Bartlett.

Gottesman, I. I., & Bertelsen, A. (1996). The legacy of German psychiatric genetics: Hindsight is always 20/20. *American Journal of Medical Genetics: Neuropsychiatric Genetics, 67,* 317–322.

Hall, L. L. (1996). *Genetics and mental illness: Evolving issues for research and society.* New York: Plenum Press.

Hanauske-Abel, H. M. (1996). Not a slippery slope or sudden subversion: German medicine and National Socialism in 1933. *British Medical Journal, 313,* 1453–63.

Leiden, J. M. (1995). Gene therapy: Promise, pitfalls, and prognosis (editorial). *New England Journal of Medicine, 333,* 871–872.

Motulsky, A. G. (1991). Ethical, legal, and social issues in human and medical genetics. *Genome, 31,* 870–865

Pross, C. (1991). *The value of the human being: Medicine in Germany, 1918–1945.* Berlin: Arztekammer.

Russell, S. J. (1997). Clinical review: Science, medicine, and the future. Gene therapy. *British Medical Journal, 315,* 1289–1292.

Sidel, V. W. (1996). The social responsibilites of health professionals: Lessons from their role in Nazi Germany. *Journal of the American Medical Association, 276,* 1679–1681.

Sram, R. J., Bulyzhenkov, V., Prikipko, L., & Christen, Y. (1991). *Ethical issues of molecular genetics in psychiatry.* Amsterdam: Springer-Verlag.

Tsuang, M. T., Faraone, S. V., & Lyons, M. J. (1993). Identification of the phenotype in psychiatric genetics. *European Archives of Psychiatry and Clinical Neuroscience, 243,* 131–142.

Wagner, J. A., & Gardner, P. (1997). Toward cystic fibrosis gene therapy. *Annual Review of Medicine, 48,* 203–216.

Weber, M. M. (1996). Ernst Rüdin, 1874–1952: A German psychiatrist and geneticist. *American Journal of Medical Genetics, 67,* 317–325.

Welch, G. H., & Burke, W. (1998). Uncertainties in genetic testing for chronic disease. *Journal of the American Medical Association, 280,* 1525–1527.

Internet Resources
for Psychiatric Genetics

Many resources are available on the Internet. New discoveries take place at a rapid pace and are updated on a regular basis online. Here we list a sample of available resources. Many of these sites will also have links to additional sites of interest.

Professional Genetics Associations on the Internet

Site	Address
American Society of Human Genetics	http://www.faseb.org/genetics/ashg/ashgmenu.htm
International Society of Psychiatric Genetics	http://www.uhmc.sunysb.edu/ispg/
American Society of Gene Therapy	http://www.asgt.org/
European Society of Human Genetics	http://www.infobiogen.fr/agora/eshg/
Behavior Genetics Association	http://www.bga.org/bga/

Internet Sites of Scientific Journals

Site	Address
American Journal of Human Genetics	http://www.ajhg.org/
Nature Genetics	http://genetics.nature.com/

Annals of Human Genetics	http://www.cup.org/Journals/JNLSCAT/hge/hge.html
Human Molecular Genetics	http://www.oup.co.uk/hmg/
American Journal of Medical Genetics	http://www.interscience.wiley.com/jpages/0148-7299/
Neuropsychiatric Genetics	http://www.interscience.wiley.com/jpages/0148-7299/
Psychiatric Genetics	http://www.chapmanhall.com/ps/default.html
Behavior Genetics	http://plenum.titlenet.com:6800/cgi/getarec?ple2000
Molecular Psychiatry	http://www.edoc.com/jrl-bin/wilma/spr.839883148.html
Genetics Journals	http://www.museum.state.il.us/isas/health/genejrnl.html

Internet Sites about the Human Genome Project

Site	Address
Human Genome Project	http://www.er.doe.gov/production/oher/hug_top.html
Ethical, Legal, and Social Implications of the Human Genome Project	http://www.kumc.edu/gec/prof/geneelsi.html
Human Genome Project Resources and Meetings	http://gdbwww.gdb.org/gdb/docs/genomic_links.html

Other Internet Sites Relevant to Psychiatric Genetics

Site	Address	Description
Primer on Human Molecular Genetics	http://www.gdb.org/Dan/DOE/intro.html	A description of molecular genetic methods for the layperson.
The Gene Letter	http://www.geneletter.org/index.htm	A newsletter on scientific and societal issues in genetics.
Information for Genetic Professionals	http://www.kumc.edu/gec/geneinfo.html	A list of useful links to genetics resources on the Internet.
GeneCards	http://bioinfo.weizmann.ac.il/cards/	An encyclopedia of genes, proteins, and diseases.

Online Mendelian Inheritance in Man	http://www3.ncbi.nlm.nih.gov/Omim/	A database listing all known genes, their products, and related diseases
NIDA Genetics Workgroup	http://www.nida.nih.gov/genetics/geneticshome.html	Information about genetic studies of drug abuse from the National Institute of Drug Abuse.
NIMH Genetics Research Branch	http://www-grb.nimh.nih.gov/grbfund.html	Information about genetic studies of drug abuse from the National Institute of Mental Health.
Genetic Linkage Analysis	http://linkage.rockefeller.edu/	Resources for the statistical analysis of genetic linkage.
Twin Methods Workshop	http://ibgwww.colorado.edu/twins96/	Information about workshops teaching twin study methodology.

Index

Note: Page numbers appearing in bold refer to definitions in the Glossary.

Abstraction ability, 65, 70
Actuarial costs, 225
Additive genes
  in oligogenic inheritance 101
  path analysis, 109–111
Adenine, 118–120, **235**
Adoptee as proband design, 39–41
Adoption studies, 39–43
  drawbacks, 44
  evaluation, 42, 43
  generalizability, 42
  in genetic epidemiology, 16
  parent as proband design, 39, 40
  in psychiatric research chain, 11,
    12
  research designs, 39–42
Affected relative pair method, **235**
Affected sib-pair method, 129–131,
  235
Agoraphobia
  behavioral inhibition risk factor,
    218, 219
  developmental continuity, 90–92
  genetic epidemiology approach,
    91, 92

Alcoholism
  path analysis, 111
  population rate, 172
  recurrence risk, families, 172
Alleles
  definition, **235**
  gel electrophoresis, 127
  in linkage analysis, 127, 128
Alpha-1-antitrypsin deficiency, 157
Alpha-7 nicotinic receptor, 202, 203
Alzheimer's disease
  causal heterogeneity, 48, 49
  family-based association study, 142
  gene discovery, 143, 144
  gene-environment interactions, 155
  genetic testing, 208, 209
  linkage analysis, 135, 136
  population-based association
    study, 139, 140
Amino acids, **235**
Amniocentesis, **235**
Amygdala, 68–70
Amyloid precursor protein
  association studies, 142
  and genetic testing, 208

Aneuploidy, **235**
Animal models, 152–155
Antisocial personality
  gene-environment interplay, 34, 35
  spectrum conditions, 62
  twin study, 33–35
Anxiety disorders
  and behavioral inhibition, 217–219
  depression comorbidity, family
    studies, 79, 80
  developmental continuity, 90–92
  genetic epidemiology approach,
    91, 92
APOE ε4 allele, 139, 140
  and genetic testing, 208, 209
  population-based association
    study, 139, 140
Association studies, 136–143
  definition, **235**
  family based, 140–143
  population based, 136–140
  replication importance, 143
Assortative mating
  and dizygotic twin studies, 38
  path analysis, 111
Attention
  and brain structure, schizophrenia,
    70
  relatives of schizophrenic patients,
    64–66, 70
Attention-deficit/hyperactivity
    disorder
  case-control family study, 16–19
  conduct disorder comorbidity, 85,
    86
  depression comorbidity, family
    studies, 78, 79, 83–86, 87–89
  developmental continuity, 90
  dopamine transporter gene,
    mouse, 154
  learning disabilities independence,
    80–82
  parental nonrandom mating, 82
  spectrum conditions, 62
Attributions, and patient education,
    192
Auditory attention

and brain structure, schizophrenia,
    70
  relatives of schizophrenic patients,
    64–66
Auditory evoked potentials, 202, 203
Autism, spectrum conditions, 62
Autoradiography, **235**
Autosomal dominance
  and genetic counseling, 170
  in single-gene transmission, 94–96
Autosomes, 118, **235**

B
Bands, chromosomal, 147–149, **235**
Bases, DNA building blocks, 118,
    235
Base-pair (bp), 120, **235**
Behavioral inhibition
  anxiety disorders predictor, 217–
    219
  physiological manifestations, 218
Berkson's bias, 74, 75
Bias, in family studies, 18, 19
Biologic property rights, 229
Biotechnology, **235**
Bipolar disorder
  adoptee as proband study, 40, 441
  depression overlap, families, 70–
    72
  linkage analysis, 123, 124, 126–
    128
  population rates, 172
  recurrence risk, families, 172
  spectrum conditions, 62
  twin studies, variance sources, 32,
    33
  two-threshold model, 106
"Blind" ratings, 19
Brain abnormalities
  and obstetric complications, schiz-
    ophrenia, 54
  relatives of schizophrenic patients,
    63–70
  schizophrenia subforms, 51, 52,
    54
Breast cancer genetic testing, 207

C

Cancer, gene therapy, 221
"Candidate genes"
   definition, 136, **236**
   in family association studies, 142
Carrier, 97, **236**
Carrier testing, **236**
Case-control method, 16–21
   bias elimination, 19
   family selection procedure, 21–25
   in family studies, 16–29
"Caseness" index, 205
Catechol-*O*-methyltransferase gene,
   152
Causal heterogeneity, 46–92
   Alzheimer's disease, 48, 49
   definition, 46, 47
   genetic studies problem, 199
Centimorgan, **236**
Centromere, 147
Chemical base, **235**
Child psychopathology
   developmental continuity, 89–92
   genetic epidemiology, 91, 92
Children, genetic testing ethics, 227,
   230
Chorionic villus sampling, **236**
Chromosome 5, schizophrenia, 151
Chromosome 6
   cytogenetic subdivisions, 147, 149
   schizophrenia linkage, 135
Chromosome 14, Alzheimer's
   disease, 135, 136
Chromosome 22q, schizophrenia,
   152
Chromosomes
   biologic characteristics, 117–124,
   236
   crossover in reproduction, 121–
   123
   cytogenetics, 146–152
   and gene identification, 120
Clinic-based studies
   diagnostic inaccuracy implications,
   23, 24
   false-positive rate, 23
   strengths and weaknesses, 22, 23
Clinical heterogeneity, 46–92, 199

Clone, **236**
Cloning, **236**
Cognitive deficits
   MRI correlation, schizophrenia,
   67–70
   relatives of schizophrenic patients,
   64–66
"Coin family" exercise, 174, 175, 178
Color blindness, linkage analysis,
   123, 124
Common (shared) environment
   antisocial personality, twins, 34
   definition, twin studies, 32
   manic-depressive psychosis, 32–33
Community-based studies (*see*
   Population-based studies)
Comorbidity, 74–89
   and Berkson's bias, 74, 75
   causes, 74–89
   clinical implications, 76
   DSM-IV approach, 74
   Epidemiologic Catchment Area
   study, 75, 76
   family history clues to, 190, 191
   family studies, 78–89
   versus hierarchical diagnostic approach, 76
   mechanisms, family studies, 80–85
   mis-diagnosis artifacts, 80
   referral artifacts, 79, 80
"Complementary base-pairs," 120,
   121
Complex inheritance, **236**
   and genetic counseling, 170
   genetic testing problem, 210–213
   mental disorders characteristic, 7,
   8
Concordant sibs, 131
Conduct disorder
   ADHD comorbidity, 85, 86
   ADHD cosegregation, 86
   spectrum conditions, 62
Confidentiality
   genetic testing ethics, 225–227
   and health insurance, 225, 226
   in pedigree construction, 167
   research participants, 231
Confirmed linkage, 134

Consanguinity, **236**
Conservative change, **236**
Conserved sequence, **236**
Contiguous gene syndromes, 152
Continuous traits
    and discontinuous psychopatholo-
        gy expression, 57, 58
    in multifactorial model, 56–58,
        102–106
    in polygenic inheritance, 102–106
"Control" probands
    in family studies, 17
    matching techniques, 24, 25
    screening criteria, 24
    selection of, 23–25
Cosegregation
    conduct disorder and ADHD, 86
    spectrum disorders, 58, 59
CpG islands, **236**
Cri du chat syndrome, 150
Cross-fostering studies, 39–41
Crossing over, 121–123, **236**
Cystic fibrosis, gene therapy, 221
Cytogenetics, 146–152
    definition, 146, **236**
    and mental illness, 150–152
Cytosine, 118–120, **237**

D
DARE program, 214, 215
Deletion mapping, **237**
Deletion mutation, 144, **237**
Demoralization, 192
Depression
    ADHD comorbidity, families, 78,
        79, 83–86, 87–89
    bipolar disorder overlap, families,
        70–72
    comorbidity odds, 75, 76
    genetic and nongenetic subtypes,
        50, 51
    population rates, 172
    recurrence risk, families, 172
    two-threshold model, 106
Developmental continuity
    anxiety disorders, 90–92
    attention-deficit/hyperactivity dis-
        order, 90

childhood and adult disorders,
    89–92
    and genetic epidemiology, 91, 92
Developmental model,
    psychopathology, 8–10
Diabetes genes, 154
Diagnosis
    and comorbidity, 74–78, 190
    family basis of, 4, 188–191
    fundamental types of inaccuracy,
        200
    in genetic counseling, 163–166
        case study, 184, 185
    genetic nosology use, 199–205
    psychiatric genetics implications,
        188–191
    reliability, 164
    sources of error, 164, 165
Diagnostic Interview for Genetic
    Studies (NIMH), 26
Diagnostic sensitivity (*see* Sensitivity,
    diagnostic)
"Diagnostician drift," 164, 165
Dinucleotide repeat, 125, 126, **237**
Diploid, **237**
Discordant sibs, linkage analysis, 131
Discrimination, genetic, 228
Dizygotic twins
    assortative mating effects, 38
    monozygotic twins comparison,
        29, 30
    schizophrenia prevalence, 30
DNA (deoxyribonucleic acid)
    biologic characteristics, 118–124,
        237
    in chromosome crossover, 121–123
    hybridization, 121
DNA fingerprinting, **237**
DNA markers
    advantages, 125
    definition, **237**
    and genetic mapping, 126
    Human Genome Project, 197, 198
    in linkage analysis, 124–136
    and method of association, 138
    Z-scores, 128, 129
DNA sequence, 125, **237**
DNA sequencing, **237**

DNA testing (*see* Genetic testing)
Dominant allele, **237**
Dominant transmission
  definition, 94
  in genetic counseling, 170
  pedigree pattern, 95, 96
Dopamine D2 receptors, 136
Dopamine transporter gene, 154
Double helix, 120, **237**
Down syndrome, 150
Drug Abuse Resistance Education
  program, 214, 215
Drug compliance, 194
DSM-IV diagnosis
  and comorbid disorders, 74, 75
  family history method diagnosis
    comparison, 27, 28
  heterogeneity problem, 199
  hierarchical diagnosis abandon-
    ment, 74, 75
Duchenne muscular dystrophy, 151
Duplication mutation, 144, **237**

E
Ecogenetics, 156–158
Educational approach
  families, 194
  patients, 191–193
Electroencephalography, 202
Electrophoresis, **237**
Emotions, and schizophrenia, 67–70
Employment discrimination, 226
Endonuclease, 125, **237**
Endophenotype, 63, **237**
Environmental influences
  brain atrophy role, schizophrenia,
    51, 52
  complex inheritance role, 7–10
  developmental model, 9, 10
  disease gene interactions, 155–158
  and genetic epidemiology, 2, 3
  mathematical models, 112
  multifactorial model, 52–55
  in patient education, 192, 193
  and primary prevention, 6, 7
  in spectrum conditions, 8
  in twins, 32–37

Enzyme, **237**
Epidemiologic Catchment Area
  study, 75, 76
Epidemiology (*see* Genetic
  epidemiology)
Epilepsy, phenotype definition, 204
Epistasis, 101, **237**
Ethical issues, 222–234
  and eugenics, 222–225
  gene therapy, 231–234
  genetic testing, 225–230
    guidelines, 226, 227
  and informed consent, 231–234
Ethical, Legal, and Social Initiative,
  224, 225
Ethnicity, 136, 137
Eugenics, 1, 222–225, **238**
Evolution, and mental illness
  prevalence, 233, 234
Exons, **238**
Experimental bias, 18, 19
Explicit matching, case-control
  studies, 25
Expressivity, **238**

F
False-negative diagnosis
  and genetic nosology, 200–205
  and phenotypic indicators, 203, 204
  types of, 200
False-positive diagnosis
  in clinic-based populations, 23, 24
  and genetic nosology, 200–205
  implications, 23
  and phenotypic indicators, 203,
    204
  sources of, 200
Familial Alzheimer's disease, 135
Family-based association studies,
  140–143
Family environment, 21
Family history
  assessment, 166
  diagnostic use, 188–191
  in genetic counseling, 166–169,
    185
  treatment use, 195

Family history method, 25–29
  advantages and disadvantages, 26,
    29
  definition, 25, 26
  diagnostic criteria, stringency, 27,
    28
  versus family study method, 29
  improvement of, procedures, 26,
    27
Family History Research Diagnostic
    Criteria interviews, 26–28,
    166
Family Interview for Genetic Studies
    (NIMH), 26, 28, 166, 167
Family studies, 16–29
  case-control method, 16–21
  clinic-based selection in, 22, 23
  comorbidity, 78–89
  control group importance, 17
  evaluation of, 21–29
  in genetic epidemiology, 16–29
  in genetic research chain, 11, 12
  population-based selection in, 22,
    23
Family study method, 25–29
Family therapy, 194, 195
First-degree relatives
  definition, 19, 20
  schizophrenia risk, 20, 21
FISH (fluorescence *in situ*
    hybridization), 151, 152, **238**

G
Galton, Francis, 222, 223
Gametes, **238**
Gel electrophoresis, 127
Gene, 119, 120, **238**
Gene detection, 116
Gene discovery, 116
Gene family, **238**
Gene map, **238**
Gene mapping, 126, **238**
Gene product, **238**
Gene testing (*see* Genetic testing)
Gene therapy, 219–221
  in cancer, 221
  in cystic fibrosis, 221

  definition, 219
  ethical issues, 231–234
  viruses in, 221
"Genetic anticipation," 145, 146
Genetic counseling, 160–188, **238**
  benefit/burden presentation, 177–
    181
  case study, 182–188
  "coin family" exercise, 174, 175,
    178
  and consultand evaluation, 173,
    176, 186, 187
  diagnostic confirmation in, 163–
    166
    case study, 184, 185
  ethical issues, 225–228
    guidelines, 226, 227
  family history assessment, 166–169
  Huntington disease, 209, 210
  nondirective nature of, 161, 162,
    181, 182
  potential impact of, 176
  probability concept presentation,
    174–176
  recurrence risk assessment/pre-
    sentation, 170–172, 176–182,
    187
  reproductive choice aspects, 176–
    182
  service availability, 160
  stages of, 160–183
  training, 160
Genetic discrimination, 228
Genetic engineering technologies,
    238
Genetic epidemiology, 15–45
  basic research designs, 15, 16
  definition, 3
  environmental factors in, 2, 3
Genetic heterogeneity, **238**
Genetic linkage (*see* Linkage analysis)
Genetic linkage map, 126, **238**
Genetic linkage mapping, **238**
Genetic markers (*see* DNA markers)
Genetic privacy laws, 227
"Genetic profiles," 230
Genetic screening, **238**

Genetic testing, 206–213
  Alzheimer's disease, 208, 209
  ethical issues, 225–230
  health insurance implications,
    225–229
  Huntington disease, 209–211
  legislation, 227, 228
  presymptomatic, 206–213
  psychiatric illness uncertainties,
    210–213
Genome, **238**
Genotype, 126, 127, **239**
Germ cells, 232, **239**
Germline gene therapy, 232–234
Germline mutation, **239**
Goodness of fit, **239**
Group matching, case-control
    studies, 25
Guanine, 118–120, **239**

H
Hallucinations, 61
Haploid, **239**
Health insurance, 225–229
  genetic testing ethics, 225–228
  legislation, 227–229
Health Insurance Portability and
    Accountability Act of 1997,
    228
Hereditary mutation, **239**
Heritability
  antisocial personality, twins, 33–35
  definition, 32
  environmental interplay, twins,
    32–37
  life cycle changes, 35
  manic-depressive psychosis, twins,
    32, 33
  spectrum disorders, 58, 59
Heterozygote, 141, **239**
Heterozygous parents, 141
Hierarchical diagnosis
  comorbidity paradigm compari-
    son, 76
  DSM approach, 74, 75
Hippocampus, schizophrenia, 67–70
Hirschsprung disease, 101

Homologies, **239**
Homologous chromosomes, **239**
Homologous structures, 153
Homozygote, 141, **239**
Homozygous parents, 141
Human Genome Project, 197, 198,
    239
Huntington disease
  genetic testing ethics, 227, 228
  linkage analysis, 117
  predictive genetic testing, 209–211
  trinucleotide repeats, 145, 146
Hybridization, **239**
Hybridize, 121, **239**
Hypercholesterolemia, 219

I
Identity by descent, **239**
Identity by state, 130, **239**
Illusions, 61
Imprinting, **239**
In vitro, **240**
Incomplete penetrance, **240**
Informants
  and comorbidity diagnosis, bias,
    78
  in family history method, 26, 27
  versus family interview informa-
    tion, 26
  psychiatric illness in, 27
Informativeness, **240**
Informed consent, 231–234
  germline gene therapy, 234
  research participation, 229, 231
Insertion mutation, 145, **240**
Intelligence genes, 233
International Classification of Diseases,
    199
Introns, **240**
Inversion mutation, 145, **240**
"Iowa 500" study, 72

J
"Junk" DNA
  definition, 119, 120
  in linkage analysis, 124–126
Juvenile myoclonic epilepsy, 204

K

Karotype, 147, **240**
Karyotyping, **240**
Kilobase (kb), **240**
"Kindling," 10
Kleinfelter syndrome, 150
Knockout, 153, 154, **240**
Kraepelin, Emil, 72, 73

L

Landmark, 147, **240**
"Latent class" states, 164
Lateral ventricles (*see* Ventricular size)
"Learned helplessness," 192
Learning disorders
  ADHD independence, family studies, 80–82
  parental nonrandom mating, 82
Liability
  definition, 104, **240**
  and patient education, 191, 192
  in spectrum conditions, 103–106
  threshold of, 104–106
Life cycle changes, heritability, 35
Life insurance, 225, 226
Likelihood, **240**
Linkage, **240**
Linkage analysis
  affected pedigree member method, 129–131
  Alzheimer's disease, 135, 136
  "caseness" index, 205
  DNA markers function in, 124–126
  examples, 134–136
  Human Genome Project contribution, 197, 198
  interpretation guidelines, 133, 134
  linkage disequilibrium studies difference, 138, 139
  "lod" score method, 131–133
  phenotypic indicators use, 201–205
  principle of, 122–124, **240**
  probability values, 133, 134
  schizophrenia, 134, 135

statistical methods, 126–136
Linkage disequilibrium
  association studies usefulness, 137, 138
  definition, 137, **240**
  linkage analysis difference, 138, 139
Linkage map, **240**
Linkage mapping, **240**
Lithium response, 193
Locus, **241**
Lod score method
  Alzheimer's disease, 135
  and complex diseases, 133
  computation, 131–133
  in linkage analysis, 131–133, **241**
Lung cancer, 155, 156

M

Mapping (*see* Gene mapping)
Marker (*see* DNA markers)
Magnetic resonance imaging, 67–70
Manic-depressive disorder (*see* Bipolar disorder)
Matching techniques, case-control studies, 24, 25
Mathematical models, 93–114
  advantages and limitations, 112–114
  overview, 107–109
  path analysis, 109–111
  in segregation analysis, 107–109
  in single-gene inheritance, 94–100, 107, 108
  twin studies contribution, 112
Maximum likelihood estimate, 132
Medical records, 29
Medication compliance, 194
Megabase (Mb), **241**
Meiosis, 144, **241**
Memory
  and brain structure, schizophrenia, 70
  relatives of schizophrenic patients, 64–66, 70
Mendelian inheritance, 94, 100, **241**
Microdeletion syndromes, 152

Microsatellites, 125, 126, **241**
Missense mutation, 145, **241**
Mitochondria, 113, **241**
Mitochondrial DNA, 113, **241**
Mitochondrial inheritance, 113, 114, **241**
"Mixed" vulnerability model, 57, 58
Mode of transmission, 94–114, **241**
Monozygotic twins
　dizygotic twins comparison, 29, 30
　environmental factors role, 3, 38
　personality development, 38
　schizophrenia prevalence, 30
　ventricular size, schizophrenia, 51, 52
Multifactorial polygenic inheritance, 101–106
　and continuous traits, 102–106
　definition, **241**
　in genetic counseling, 171, 172
　"normal distribution," 102, 103
　in patient education, 191, 192
　schizophrenia, 52–55
　spectrum conditions, 55–58
　and vulnerability, 56–58
Mutation, 119, 144–146, **241**

N
Nature-nurture debate, 3
Nazi eugenics abuses, 223, 224
"Negative" symptoms, 60, 61
Neurodegeneration, 10
Neurodevelopmental factors, 9, 10
Neurofibromatosis type 1, 47
Neuropsychological tests
　MRI correlation, schizophrenia, 67–70
　relatives of schizophrenic patients, 64–66
Newborn screening, **241**
Nicotinic receptors, schizophrenia, 202, 203
Nitrogenous base (*see* Base)
Nonadditive genetic effects, 109–111
Non-Mendelian inheritance
　definition, 100
　mitochondria, 113, 114
Nonrandom mating, 82, 87, 88
Nonsense mutation, 145, **241**
Nonshared environment
　antisocial personality, twins, 34
　definition, twin studies, 32
　manic-depressive psychosis, 32, 33
　path analysis, 109–111
Nosology, genetic, 199–205
Nucleotide, 125, **241**
Nucleus, **241**

O
Obstetric complications, 54
Oculomotor dysfunction, 203, 204
Oligogenic inheritance, 100, 101, **242**
Oncogenes, 153

P
P arm, 147, **242**
P50 wave, 202, 203
Panic disorder
　behavioral inhibition risk factor, 218, 219
　developmental continuity, 90–92
　genetic counseling, risk presentation, 176–181
　genetic epidemiology approach, 91, 92
　spectrum conditions, 62
　survival advantages, gene dosage, 233, 234
Paranoia, and study participation, 25
Parent as proband design, 39, 40
Participation rates, family studies, 25
Paternal half-sibling studies, 39, 41, 42
Path analysis, 109–111
　definition, 109, 110, **242**
　family data, 110, 111
Path coefficients, 110, **242**
Patient education, 191–193
Patient's rights, 229
PCR (polymerase chain reaction), **242**

Pedigree
  definition, **242**
  in genetic counseling, 167–169,
    184
    case study, 184
  graphic representations, 96, 98,
    99, 167–169
  mathematical models, 108, 109
  in single-gene inheritance, 94–99
  symbols in, 167–169
Penetrance, 107, 108, **242**
Personality, monozyotic twins, 38
Personality spectrum disorders, 60,
  61
Phage, **242**
Pharmacogenetics, 193
Phenocopy
  causal heterogeneity, 48
  definition, 48, **242**
Phenotype
  definition, 204, 205, **242**
  in linkage analysis, 201–205
Phenylketonuria
  gene-environment interplay, 36,
    37, 156, 157
  medical interventions, 219–221
Phobias
  developmental continuity, 90–92
  genetic epidemiology approach,
    91, 92
Physical map, **242**
Pleiotropy, **242**
Point mutations, 145
Polygenic disorders, **242** (*see also*
  Multifactorial polygenic
  inheritance)
Polymerase chain reaction, **242**
Polymorphism, **242**
Polymorphism information content,
  242
Population-based studies, 136–140
  Alzheimer's disease success, 139,
    140
  diagnostic inaccuracy implications,
    23
  ethnic group factors, 136, 137

and linkage disequilibrium, 137–
  139
  strengths and weaknesses, 22, 23
Population isolates, 137
Positional cloning, 117, **242**
"Positive symptoms," 60, 61
Precursor syndromes, 77
Predictive genetic tests, **243**
Pregnancy, in neurodevelopmental
  model, 9
Prenatal diagnosis, 206, **243**
Presenilin genes, discovery, 143, 144
Presymptomatic diagnosis, 206–213
  ethics, 225–228
  future prospects, 206–213
Prevention programs, 213–219
  anxiety disorders, 217–219
  primary versus secondary, 213,
    214
  psychosocial and medical services,
    215
  schizophrenia, 215–217
  selective versus universal, 214, 215
Primary prevention, 6, 7, 213, 214
Probability, 174–176, **243**
Probability values, lod scores, 133,
  134
Probands
  in case-control family studies, 16–
    21
  definition, **243**
  matching techniques, 24, 25
  selection of, 21–25
Prodromal conditions, 56
Promoter, **243**
Proofreader genes, **243**
Protein, 119, **243**
"Psychiatric genetic nosology," 199–
  205
Psychosis, and kindling, 10
Psychosis not otherwise specified,
  59, 60
Purine, **243**

Q
Q arm, 147, **243**
Quantitative trait, **243**

R

Recessive allele
  definition, 94, 95, **243**
  pedigree pattern, 95, 97, 98
Recombinant DNA molecules, **243**
Recombinant DNA technologies, **243**
Recombination, **243**
Recombination fraction, 132, 135, **243**
Recurrence risk
  empirical estimates, 170, 171
  in genetic counseling, 170–172, 176–182
    case example, 185, 187
  multifactorial polygenic model, 171, 172
  population risk comparison, 178, 179
  presentation of, 176–182, 187
Referral artifacts
  comorbidity, 79, 80, 86
  conduct disorder and ADHD co-morbidity, 86
  depression and ADHD comorbidity, 87, 88
Regulatory regions, **243**
Relatives
  of bipolar patients, 70–72
  of depressed patients, 70–73
  diagnostic use, 188–191
  of schizophrenia patients, 63–70, 72, 73
    neurobiology, 63–70
Reliability, diagnostic, 164
Repeat expansion detection, 146
Repeat sequences, **244**
Replication, **244**
Reporter bias, 78
Reproductive cells, **244**
Reproductive choice, 176–182
Research participation
  confidentiality, 225, 226
  informed consent, 231
  patient's rights, 229
Resolution, **244**
Restriction enzymes, 125, **244**

Restriction fragment length polymorphism (RFLP), 125, 127, **244**
Reverse genetics, 117, **244**
Risk (*see also* Liability; Recurrence risk)
  family concerns, 5
  vulnerability relationship, 30

S

Schizoaffective disorders, 59, 60
Schizophrenia
  adoption studies, 40
  brain atrophy, 51, 52, 54, 63–70
  cross-fostering study, 40, 41
  cytogenetic abnormalities, 150–152
  genetic and non-genetic subforms, 51, 52
  genetic counseling, 176–188
    case study, 183–188
    risk presentation, 176–182
  genetic nosology, 201–205
  genetic risk, relatives, 20, 21
  genetic subtypes, 53, 54
  and kindling, 10
  linkage analysis, 135, 202–205
  multifactorial theory, 52–56, 102–106
  neurobiological correlates, families, 63–70
  paternal half-sibling study, 41, 42
  path analysis, 110, 111
  phenotype definition, linkage analysis, 202–205
  polygenic inheritance, 103–106
  population-based versus clinic-based studies, 22, 23
  prevention programs, 213–217
    and childhood predictors, 215–217
  recurrence risk, families, 172
  spectrum disorders, 55–62, 103–106
  survival advantages, gene dosage, 233
  twin studies, 30

Schizophrenia families
  MRI data, 67–70
  neurobiology, 63–70
  neuropsychological tests, 64–66
  stability over time, 66
Schizotypal personality disorder, 61
Screening artifacts, 77
Second-degree relatives
  definition, 19, 20
  schizophrenia risk, 20, 21
Secondary disorders, 78
Secondary prevention, 214
Segregation, **244**
Segregation analysis, 106–109
  definition, 106
  in genetic research chain, 11, 12
  mathematical models, 106–109
  in psychiatric disorders, limita-
    tions, 109
Selective prevention programs
  definition, 214
  schizophrenia, 215–217
Self-esteem, and therapy, 191–193
Semistructured interviews, 26–28, 166
Sensitivity, diagnostic
  in clinic-based studies, 23, 24
  implications of errors, 23
  in population-based studies, 23
Sensory gating, schizophrenia, 202,
  203
Separation anxiety
  adult anxiety risk factor, 91
  and behavioral inhibition, 218
Sequence, **244**
Sequence tagged site, **244**
Sequencing, **244**
Severe combined immune
  deficiency, 220
Sex chromosomes, 97, 118, **244**
Sex-linked disorders
  pedigree pattern, 97, 99
  single-gene inheritance, 97–100
Shared environment
  antisocial personality, twins, 34
  definition, twin studies, 32
  manic-depressive psychosis, 32, 33
  path analysis, 109–111

Shy children, 217–219
Sib-pair method
  in linkage analysis, 129–131, 134
  suggestive linkage probabilities,
    134
Sickle cell anemia, 233
Significant linkage, 134
Single-gene disorder, 94–100, 107,
  108, **244**
Single major gene, **244**
Smoking, gene interactions, 155, 156
Social phobia
  developmental continuity, 90–92
  genetic epidemiology approach,
    91, 92
Somatic cell gene therapy, 232
Somatic cells, **244**
Somatic mutation, **244**
Spectrum disorders, 55–63
  definition, 7, 8
  genes and environment interac-
    tions, 8
  identification of, 58–63
  liability, 103–106
  and multifactorial vulnerability
    model, 55–58
  neurobiology, schizophrenia, 63–
    70
  outcome versus precursor distinc-
    tion, 62
  and polygenic inheritance, 103–
    106
  schizophrenia, 55–62, 103–106
Statistical methods, linkage analysis,
  126–136
Statistical significance, 18
Stigmatization, 177, 191
Suggestive linkage, 134

T
Tandem repeat sequences, 125, **245**
Telomeres, **245**
Temperament (*see* Behavioral
  inhibition)
Teratogen, **245**
Thalamus, 67–70
Therapeutic nihilism, 191–193

Third-degree relatives
    definition, 19, 20
    schizophrenia risk, 20, 21
Threshold model, 56, 57
Thymine, 118–120, **245**
Tourette syndrome, 62
Transgenic organism, 153, **245**
Translocation mutation
    in cytogenetics, 150
    definition, 144, 150, **245**
Transmission disequilibrium test, **245**
Trinucleotide repeats
    and "genetic anticipation," 145
    Huntington disease, 145, 146
Trisomy, 150, **245**
Twin studies, 29–39
    antisocial personality, 33–35
    drawbacks, 44
    evaluation, 37–39
    generalization of, 37, 38
    genetic and environment inter-
        play, 32–37
    in genetic epidemiology, 16
    in genetic research chain, 11, 12
    mathematical models, 112
    ventricular size, schizophrenia, 51,
        52

U
Unique environment (*see* Nonshared
    environment)
Universal preventive programs, 214,
    215

V
VAPSE, 146, **245**
Variable number of tandem repeats,
    125, 126
Velo-cardio-facial syndrome, 152

Ventricular size
    genetic versus nongenetic schizo-
        phrenia, 51, 52
    and obstetric complications, 54
    relatives of schizophrenic patients,
        67–69
    schizophrenia subforms, 51, 52
Verbal memory
    and brain structure, schizophrenia,
        70
    relatives of schizophrenic patients,
        64–66, 70
Virus
    definition, **245**
    in gene transfer, 221
Vulnerability
    continuum of, 56–58
    definition, 30
    family history clues, 190
    "mixed model," 57, 58
    multifactorial model, 31, 56–58

W
Working memory, 66

X
X chromosome, 118, **245**
X-linked disease
    bipolar disorder, linkage analysis,
        123
    definition, 97, **245**
    pedigree pattern, 97, 99

Y
Y chromosome, 118, **245**

Z
Z-score, 128, 129
Zygosity determination, 37